CAMBRIDGE LIBRARY COLLECTION

Books of enduring scholarly value

History of Medicine

It is sobering to realise that as recently as the year in which *On the Origin of Species* was published, learned opinion was that diseases such as typhus and cholera were spread by a 'miasma', and suggestions that doctors should wash their hands before examining patients were greeted with mockery by the profession. The Cambridge Library Collection reissues milestone publications in the history of Western medicine as well as studies of other medical traditions. Its coverage ranges from Galen on anatomical procedures to Florence Nightingale's common-sense advice to nurses, and includes early research into genetics and mental health, colonial reports on tropical diseases, documents on public health and military medicine, and publications on spa culture and medicinal plants.

Medical Notes on Climate, Diseases, Hospitals, and Medical Schools, in France, Italy, and Switzerland

Having trained in Edinburgh as a surgeon and served aboard Royal Navy vessels, Sir James Clark (1788–1870) developed a particular interest in the spread of the tuberculosis pandemic in Europe. A licentiate of the Royal College of Physicians from 1826, and elected to the Royal Society in 1832, he became a trusted physician and friend to Queen Victoria and Prince Albert. This early work of 1820 was based on his first-hand knowledge of the treatment of tuberculosis in southern Europe as well as the effects of climate on the disease. Among his tubercular patients in Italy around this time was the poet John Keats (who would succumb in 1821). Also reissued in this series are Clark's *Treatise on Pulmonary Consumption* (1835), his *Memoir of John Conolly* (1869), and *The Influence of Climate in the Prevention and Cure of Chronic Diseases* (1829), a development of aspects of the present work.

Cambridge University Press has long been a pioneer in the reissuing of out-of-print titles from its own backlist, producing digital reprints of books that are still sought after by scholars and students but could not be reprinted economically using traditional technology. The Cambridge Library Collection extends this activity to a wider range of books which are still of importance to researchers and professionals, either for the source material they contain, or as landmarks in the history of their academic discipline.

Drawing from the world-renowned collections in the Cambridge University Library and other partner libraries, and guided by the advice of experts in each subject area, Cambridge University Press is using state-of-the-art scanning machines in its own Printing House to capture the content of each book selected for inclusion. The files are processed to give a consistently clear, crisp image, and the books finished to the high quality standard for which the Press is recognised around the world. The latest print-on-demand technology ensures that the books will remain available indefinitely, and that orders for single or multiple copies can quickly be supplied.

The Cambridge Library Collection brings back to life books of enduring scholarly value (including out-of-copyright works originally issued by other publishers) across a wide range of disciplines in the humanities and social sciences and in science and technology.

Medical Notes on Climate, Diseases, Hospitals, and Medical Schools, in France, Italy, and Switzerland

Comprising an Inquiry into the Effects of a Residence in the South of Europe, in Cases of Pulmonary Consumption

JAMES CLARK

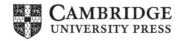

CAMBRIDGE
UNIVERSITY PRESS

CAMBRIDGE
UNIVERSITY PRESS

University Printing House, Cambridge, CB2 8BS, United Kingdom

Published in the United States of America by Cambridge University Press, New York

Cambridge University Press is part of the University of Cambridge.
It furthers the University's mission by disseminating knowledge in the pursuit of
education, learning and research at the highest international levels of excellence.

www.cambridge.org
Information on this title: www.cambridge.org/9781108064347

© in this compilation Cambridge University Press 2013

This edition first published 1820
This digitally printed version 2013

ISBN 978-1-108-06434-7 Paperback

MEDICAL NOTES

ON

CLIMATE, DISEASES, HOSPITALS, AND MEDICAL SCHOOLS,

IN

FRANCE, ITALY, AND SWITZERLAND;

COMPRISING

AN INQUIRY INTO THE EFFECTS

OF

A RESIDENCE IN THE SOUTH OF EUROPE,

IN CASES OF

PULMONARY CONSUMPTION,

AND ILLUSTRATING

𝔗𝔥𝔢 𝔓𝔯𝔢𝔰𝔢𝔫𝔱 𝔖𝔱𝔞𝔱𝔢 𝔬𝔣 𝔐𝔢𝔡𝔦𝔠𝔦𝔫𝔢

IN THOSE COUNTRIES.

BY JAMES CLARK, M. D.

LONDON:

PRINTED FOR T. AND G. UNDERWOOD, 32, FLEET-STREET ;
SOLD ALSO BY T. VIGURS, PENZANCE : AND
T. BESLEY, JUN. 223, HIGH-
STREET, EXETER.

1820.

T. VIGURS, PRINTER, PENZANCE.

Dedication.

—◆◈◆—

Sir,

If the following work had received all the improvement of which it is susceptible, and, through means of much more time and study than have been bestowed on it, had attained a degree of value and interest proportionate to the great importance of the subjects of which it treats, there is no individual to whom I should have been so proud of submitting it as to yourself, whose professional talents, equalled only by your opportunities of acquiring practical knowledge, must have constituted you the best judge of its merits: in its present imperfect condition I can only offer it to you as a sincere though humble testimony of my respect and esteem.

I have the honour to be,

Sir,

Your much obliged and faithful humble Servant,

THE AUTHOR.

Rome, Nov. 16, 1819.

PREFACE.

Letter addressed to John Forbes, M. D., Secretary of the Royal Geological Society of Cornwall, and Physician to the Penzance Dispensary.

DEAR SIR,

I HEREWITH, at length, transmit you the concluding portion of my notes on the Climate, Diseases, and Medical Practice of those places on the Continent which I have hitherto visited; and when I take a review of them thus finished, and such as they are to meet the eye of the Public, I confess to you that the sense of their unworthiness, which I originally urged as a motive for my declining to publish them when this measure was first suggested by yourself, presses on my mind more than ever. The die is however now cast, and all that remains for me, thus placed upon the stage, is to make the best excuse I can, first, for my appearance there at all, and secondly, for the indifferent part which I am apprehensive my Auditors and Judges may consider me as performing. I have therefore to request that you will affix this Letter by way of Preface to my Book, without addition or diminution.

From the period of my first coming on the Continent, two years ago, it certainly was my intention
to take advantage of the opportunities that might be
offered me of collecting information respecting the
climate, diseases, and medical practice of the places
which I might visit, as well with the view of cheering
hours, which I had reason to apprehend (from circumstances that need not here be mentioned) might
hang rather heavy on my hands, as from the desire
of professional improvement, and, partly also, I will
confess, with the intention of eventually laying the
fruits of my observations before the Public, should they
ever reach that degree of maturity and importance
that might warrant and justify such a proceeding.

The whole of the above mentioned period, with
the exception of six weeks last autumn which I spent
in England, was past at one or other of the places
noticed in the notes. The circumstances under which
I visited these different places were very various in
as far as regards the time and relative facilities
allowed for observation : in some places my stay was
very short, and the facilities of observation considerable ; in others these circumstances were reversed,
and in some they were otherwise, and still more un-
favourably combined. I mention this as acccounting
for the great inequality that will be found in the
quantity of information respecting different places,
and especially as an excuse for the great meagerness
in my account of some of them. I think it however
right to say, that, as all the matter contained in the
work was collected on the spot, and from equally
authentic sources, I consider the accounts of *all* the

places mentioned as equally entitled to credit and consideration. At least the only limitation that seems to me at all necessary to be made to this general statement, is, in as far as regards the *climate* of particular places : as a personal knowledge of this can only be attained by a residence of some considerable duration, I think it proper to declare that the only places at which I consider my stay to have been sufficiently ample for this purpose, are Marseilles, Hieres, Nice, Lausanne, and Rome.

My notes, thus collected, I brought to England with me in September, fully aware of their scantiness and imperfection ; conscious that they must appear to those unacquainted with the particular circumstances under which they were written, as disproportionate in point of value to the very considerable time during which they were collected, and never dreaming of submitting them, in their present state of imperfection, to the tribunal of the public. On showing them however to yourself, and some other of my friends, your arguments and persuasions at length overcame my scruples ; and the work now submitted to the reader, consists of the materials then collected, only somewhat more formally arranged, and of a few additional remarks obtained during my late journey from Paris to this city.

Having thus thrown the responsibility of my appearance before the public on your shoulders, it would, perhaps, be but fair to make *you* answerable for the degree of credit hazarded by the proceeding ; but, as I fear that the awarders of the doom that awaits this production at the critical tribunal, may

be rather inclined to visit its sins on the real parent,
I think it necessary to state, in a few words, the principal reasons that have weighed with me in yielding
to your suggestions.

In the first place, with regard to the investigation
of the subject to which almost the whole of **Part First**
is devoted—viz. *the influence of Southern Climates
on Consumption;*—the inquiry is of such immense
importance at present, when this disease is so alarm-
ingly prevalent, and when its victims crowd in such
numbers to the countries treated of, that the only
objection I could have to the publication of my
remarks, was the prospect I had of greatly enlarging
them, by additional experience, at no very distant
period, As, however, many circumstances might
occur to prevent the accomplishment of this hope, it
has been considered better to communicate without
further delay, information, which, though not extensive, may yet be useful, than to risk, for the sake of
possible improvement or personal credit, the occurrence of a contingency, which, after all, might pos-
sibly never be attained.

With respect to the subject of **Part Second,** (the
account, namely, of *Hospitals and Medical Schools)*
although the latter consideration is equally applicable,
the former is certainly not so : as perhaps compen-
sating the want of this it may, however, be urged that
the *novelty* of much of the matter comes in as an ar-
gument sufficiently exculpatory :—since it must be

allowed that very little information respecting several
of the institutions noticed in this part, has of late
years been laid before the English medical public.

In respect to the work itself, I beg it to be expli-
citly understood that I wish it to be considered literally what it is designated, namely, as detached
NOTES on a few of the very numerous and important
objects presented to my view ; those I have not
touched on being, if not equally interesting, at least
sufficiently so to deserve the notice of the medical
observer, and ought to claim the attention of the professed traveller, and form an essential part of a treatise composed on the subject of these desultory notices.
As far as regards the facts and the opinions contained
in these notes, I, of course, must submit to see them
tried by their intrinsic value, but I am unwilling to
be blamed for omissions (that must be every where
perceptible) which I pretend not to be ignorant of,
—and which, perhaps, are inevitable,—with equal
severity as if I came before the public, with the pretensions of a professed traveller, or the responsibility
justly attached to the author of a formal treatise.

Whatever be the decision of my brethren on my
little work I certainly shall not regret that I submitted
it to their inspection, and still less, that I composed
it ; the consciousness of right motives, and the feel-
ing of, at least, individual improvement, during the
process of its composition, will make me amends for
a worse reception of it than even my humble opinion
of its value leads me to anticipate: at all events it
will be useful to myself as a sort of text-book for

b

future observations of a like nature, and as a basis
whereon, I hope, more extensive opportunities may
enable me to rear a superstructure at once more creditable to myself, more commensurate with the importance of the subject, and more worthy the attention of the public.

After all these apologies, explanations, and pro-
mises, (the extent of which, I fear, may seem to argue
in the Author higher pretensions than his words
avow,) allow me, before concluding, to thank you,
my dear sir, for all the trouble you have so kindly
undertaken for my sake.

Much of what is contained in my Essay was, you
well know, originally communicated to yourself by
letter ; and when I consider this circumstance,
together with the share you had in my first visiting
the Continent, the encouragement you have given
me to make my observations public, and your kindness in superintending their publication (without
which they certainly could not have now appeared,)
it is but justice to acknowledge, that, if my little
work contain any useful information, to you the
public is chiefly indebted for it.

In thus publicly thanking you for this new instance
of your kindness, you must allow me the additional
gratification of acknowledging how highly I prize
the friendship which has so long united us, a friendship which commenced with our school-boy days,
cheered us through our maturer studies, and which
will still continue, I trust, to be in future, as here-

tofore, esteemed by us both, as none of the least
blessings of this life.

That you may long continue to enjoy the reputation and esteem which talents and virtues deserve,
will ever be the warmest wish of

DEAR SIR,

Your affectionate Friend,

JAMES CLARK.

Rome, November 16, 1819.

Note by the Editor.

—

To those who have read Dr. Carter's Book, recently published, entitled " A Short Account of some of the principal Hospitals of France, Italy, Switzerland and the Netherlands, with remarks upon the Climate, and diseases of those Countries " it is unnécèssary to say that the Author has by no means exhausted any of the subjects treated of by him, and that he has thus left room for the observations of succeeding writers even on those places which he has noticed Accordingly I think it will be found that nothing contained in Dr. Carter's Book could have justified the suppression of any part of Dr. Clark's. In some points their observations correspond, but, in general, they appear to have pursued different lines of enquiry.

It is scarcely necessary to mention that almost the whole of Dr. Clark's notes were written before Dr. Carter's work issued from the press.

J. F.

CONTENTS.

PART FIRST.

PART SECOND.

PART FIRST.

NOTES

ON THE

CLIMATE AND DISEASES

OF THE

SOUTH of FRANCE, ITALY,

AND

SWITZERLAND.

——— Aliis alius locus est inimicus
Partibus, ac membris : varius concinnat id aer.
Lucret; De Rer. Nat. Lib. vi, 1. 1115.

PART FIRST.

ON CLIMATE AND DISEASES.

HAVING visited most of the Places in the SOUTH OF FRANCE and ITALY, which have been recommended as eligible residences for the Consumptive Patients annually sent abroad from our own Island, in the hope of finding in those milder Climes a restoration of health, or at least an alleviation of their complaints ; and having kept accurate notes on the climate, and its effects upon disease, as well from my own observation as from that of the resident Medical Men, I have ventured, not without much diffidence, to lay the following observations before the Public. I have been induced to do this, in the hope that they may prove of some utility to the very interesting class of my Countrymen, for whom they are chiefly intended ; and perhaps, also, assist the

A

English Physician, who has not had the advantage of visiting these places, and who may be of opinion that such a change of climate is useful, in directing his patients in the choice of a residence. If this hope shall be realized, the intention of this publication will be quite fulfilled, and I shall be more than repaid for any trouble I may have had in collecting the remarks it contains.

My attention was particularly called to the subject of this Essay, on first going to the Continent, from knowing that the minds of English Practitioners were generally undecided on the propriety of sending Consumptive Patients abroad, and when they were sent, what particular situation deserved a preference over the others. I had abundan proof of this in the contradictory advices, which I found some of our most celebrated Physicians had given to the invalids I met with; some of these being sent to the South of France indiscriminately, others being recommended to MARSEILLES, others to HIERES, many to NICE; while not a few of their medical advisers candidly avowed their ignorance of the most desirable residence, and left the choice to the discretion of their patients.

That such discrepancy of opinion, and consequent indecision, should still exist on this
point, after the number of English Medical Men
that have visited these places, since Doctor
SMOLLET first called the attention of our Countrymen to NICE, is a matter of much surprize.
The subject, however, it must be owned, is one
of no little difficulty ; and, I doubt not, many
medical men have been deterred from making
their opinions public, from a belief that their
own experience had been far too limited to
enable them to speak with decision ;—a circumstance which is the more to be regretted, as it
is only by the united observations of many, that
the matter can be finally settled. Of the
medical men who have spoken of these climates,
—some in favour, others against them,—the
generality have been contented with stating
their opinions without giving us the grounds
upon which they were founded ; while some
have written from theoretical notions alone,
without any experience of the places they
describe :—trusting to the latitude, the vicinity
of mountains, and so forth. That the only
effect of such vagueness should be to excite
doubt and indecision, is not to be wondered at.

During the last forty years, our knowledge
on this point, seems to have advanced but one
step—from error to uncertainty.   At the
commencement of the period just stated,
MONTPELIER was the situation almost invariably recommended in cases of consumption,
and continued to be so for many years ; so that
its name came to be very commonly applied
as a characteristic epithet to places supposed
to be particularly healthy.   The climate of
Montpelier is, nevertheless, now generally admitted to be a very improper one during the
winter for such patients ; and no English Physician thinks of sending such invalids there at
present.   A stronger instance than this can
scarcely be adduced, of the slow progress of
our knowledge in such matters, or of the impropriety of trusting to the information obtained
from vague reports of the latitude, &c., without
taking into consideration the many other circumstances of the locality, which are, at least,
equally important in enabling us to decide on
its actual or relative goodness, as a station for
individuals affected with particular diseases.
Of these other circumstances, not the least seldom overlooked is the one most important of
all, namely, the knowledge derived from expe-

rience, which, after all our meteorological observations and pathological reasoning, must
continue to be our best guide in this, as in other
instances.

That the observations contained in the following pages will fill up the blank in our information on this subject, I am far from believing;
yet I am not without hopes that they may be
found useful in this way, and that they will
serve as a ground-work for future observers of
more extensive experience, and with abilities
and leisure more fitted for the task.

In order to avoid as much as possible some
of the causes to which I have attributed the
present unsettled state of opinion on the subject
of this essay, I shall endeavour to be as me-
thodical as the nature of my subject, and the
extent of my information will admit.

Taking it for granted that my readers are
unacquainted with the local situation of the
places to be mentioned, I shall give in the
ensuing remarks, first, a short topographical
account of each, (confining myself, however,
strictly to those circumstances which appear

to me immediately connected with its locality
in a medical point of view) ; secondly, observations on its climate ; and thirdly, remarks
on the diseases in which it seems useful or injurious, founded on these observations, and on a
knowledge of the ailments to which the Inhabitants are most liable. To these will be occasionally added a few remarks on the present
state of medical practice, as far as sufficient
information could be gained on that point.

The medical reader will thus be put in
possession of information sufficient to enable
him in some measure to form his own judgment,
unbiassed by any opinions which I may venture
to give.

MARSEILLES.

The order in which the places are described is a matter of no consequence. I begin with Marseilles as the first which I visited. Here I found several Consumptive Patients, and among others one in whom I felt particularly interested. This gentleman had been sent thither from England to pass the winter; but that a more improper residence could scarcely have been selected, it will not, I think, be difficult to show.

Marseilles is a large handsome City, containing nearly 100,000 Inhabitants. It is built upon a gentle declivity, sloping into a fine bay of the Mediterranean, and facing the northwest. The lower part of the town almost surrounds one of the finest harbours that can be imagined. Behind the city, at the distance of several miles, rises a ridge of high rugged mountains, which, like most of those in Provence, are of a most unseemly aspect, except perhaps, to the eye of the Geologist ;—presenting nothing but a rugged and barren mass of

B

rock for about two thirds of their height. These
mountains form a semicircular sweep termi-
nating in the sea on each side of the town,
which they encompass on all sides, except
towards the north-west.

The whole space between the town and
the mountains is divided into small patches by
high white walls, inclosing the country-houses
(bastides), used as summer residences by
the wealthy Marseillois. The roads leading
from the town to these houses, (almost of
sufficient number to form another Marseilles,)
are narrow, and from the arid nature of the soil,
generally dusty. The walls are high, and frequently overhung with olive-trees, so that the
invalid who leaves the town in hopes of enjoying a country ride, and something like country
scenery, finds himself wholly disappointed ; his
view being entirely confined to the winding
paths, if we except an occasional glimpse of
the surrounding country-houses, or of the tops
of the uninteresting mountains just mentioned.
Indeed it may be said there is no *country* about
Marseilles for the invalid residing there,—a
defect of no small importance to that class of
individuals.

But the great evil of Marseilles, as a winter
residence, to the consumptive, or those liable
to inflammatory affections of the chest, is the
frequency and force of the dry cold northerly
winds, to which, during that season, it is particularly subject, and to the full influence of
which its northerly aspect exposes it in a peculiar manner. The effect of these winds, the
most frequent and violent of which is the north-
west,* termed by the Inhabitants the *Mistral*,—
is to produce a very great and often very sudden
alteration of temperature. This is severely felt
by the Inhabitants themselves, (the surface
being probably relaxed, and rendered particularly sensible, by the preceding heats,) and
on many occasions, cannot be guarded against
by the most cautious invalid. The influence of
this wind in sinking the Thermometer is by no
means in proportion to its effects on the living
body. In this respect, indeed, the indications
of the thermometer form a very incorrect test
of the character of a climate; a circumstance
which, from being too little attended to, has
been another source of error in forming our
opinions of the mildness or severity of any given

* The prevalence of this wind will be seen by a reference to the
Meteorological Tables for Marseilles in the Appendix.—It frequently
blows with violence for several days together.

district. This has been well remarked by the
learned author of the " Essay on the Medical
Effects of Climates," and I have had frequent
occasion to verify the truth of the observation.
" The simple indications of a thermometer, (he
says) however accurately they may be observed,
in the most unexceptionable exposure, by no
means afford a correct test of the temperature,
as it affects the human system : nor is it possible to express the modifications produced by
wind and moisture, even supposing them to be
easily known, by any numerical measure, which
shall be applicable to every relative situation
of the individual ; I have known an atmosphere
at 65°, with a thick fog, and a very little wind
from n. e. appear, to a person taking moderate
exercise, most oppressively sultry ; although a
person sitting long still, might have felt the same
air uncomfortably cold."*

On the 24th of november, the mistral blew
with considerable violence, and, to the feelings,
was extremely cold; yet the thermometer,
which, the day before, at 2 p. m. had stood at
55°, at the same hour on this day, had only
sunk to 48°,—an effect on the thermometer

* Essay on Climates in Dr. Young's Treatise on Consumptive
Diseases, p. 83.

certainly by no means equivalent to that produced on the living body. During the prevalence of this wind, which is generally accompanied with a clear cloudless atmosphere, the
sun is often very powerful ; and, exposed to
it, in a sheltered situation, the invalid may enjoy
a very high temperature ; but this only makes
him feel, with greater severity, the chilling
blast, the moment he leaves this sort of artificial climate.

From this account of the climate of Marseilles,
we might, perhaps, rest satisfied as to the
effects to be expected from it in pulmonary
consumption ; but I shall adduce evidence still
more positive, and which, I think, will set at
rest for ever the question of the eligibility of
this place as a residence for the consumptive.*
In the Annual Report of the Diseases of Marseilles, read before the Royal Medical Society
of that place, in 1816, by Dr. Segaud the Secretary, are the following remarks, which I
translate from the original: " The natives of
the country, as well as strangers coming to

---

* It is scarcely necessary to remark that a climate, the Inhabitants
of which are particularly liable to any disease, and where strangers
must be exposed to the causes that produce it, is as improper as a
preventive, as it would be as a *curative* of the same disease in strangers.

reside here, who have *well-formed chests,* and who live temperately, attain to a great age. —The most frequent endemial diseases are Phthisis Pulmonalis, Eruptions, Schirrus Uteri, &c. The first of these (Phthisis Pulmonalis) which is often hereditary, and sometimes acquired through the little care taken to avoid the causes which give rise to it, produces inconceivable ravages among the younger part of the population."*

From the same Physician, who kindly gave me written answers to my different queries on the climate and diseases of Marseilles, I chiefly obtained the following additional information : †
The general character of the climate of Marseilles is dry and variable, and, as we have just seen, destructive to patients affected with consumption. It is, indeed, one of the towns of France, in which this disease is the most preva-

---

* " La premiere," &c , " fait des ravages inouis en moissonnant la plus belle jeunesse." Exposé des travaux de la societé de Medecine de Marseille pendant l'anné medicale de 1816, par M. Segaud Secretaire General, p. 14.

† This plan of getting written answers I invariably adopted, and it is the only way of procuring accurate information on such subjects. A man in conversation may give incorrect information unintentionally from not reflecting sufficiently, but a person generally reflects a little before he commits his answers to paper.

lent. Females from fourteen to eighteen years
of age are its most frequent victims. In some
cases it runs its course with great rapidity; in
others the patient lives six, eight, and even
twelve months, and, in a small proportion of
cases, lingers for years. It attacks most frequently during autumn and winter. Dr. S.
believes it invariably fatal. Scrophula attacking
external parts of the body, is a rare disease
at Marseilles. Pleurisy, and Catarrh, are very
frequent. Cancer and Cutaneous Diseases are
common. Diseases requiring a dry climate,
and not injured by keen cold winds, may
expect to derive benefit from a residence at
Marseilles. In the cure of intermittent fevers
I was informed it is particularly favourable;
cases, which in other places had resisted the
use of every remedy, getting well here without the use of any medicine.

The above evidence on the climate of
Marseilles, I think will be considered conclusive. The part of the town most sheltered from
the mistral is the northern side of the harbour.
Here, or perhaps in some of the country-houses
could one be found with the ground rising to
the north-ward of it, a consumptive patient

under *the necessity* of passing the winter at this
place, would find the greatest safety. Those
who can choose their climate should not be
found at Marseilles after the month of october.

My opportunities of observing the state of
medical practice in this place were not very
numerous. They have a respectable Medical
Society, of which the celebrated Professor
Foderé was one of the founders. They publish
a small report of their proceedings annually.
Attached to the Society is a small Museum of
wax-work, anatomical, or rather pathological
preparations. They are mostly illustrative of
diseases, and upon the whole, are accurate
representations. The General Hospital is
large, but badly planned, badly lighted and
ventilated, and, above all, not very clean.
At the time of my visit there were no cases particularly deserving remark. In a small close
room I found an English sailor : he had been
three months confined there for rheumatism,
and the principal remedies, he told me, had
been warm poultices to the affected joints !
It may be worth while here to remark a
circumstance affecting the practice of medicine
at Marseilles. How far it exists in other parts
of France, I have not been able to learn, but

wherever it does exist, it cannot fail to have a considerable influence in deadening professional enterprize and rendering practice inert. The circumstance I allude to, is a very general prejudice which exists towards any physician, who loses a patient, by the family of that patient. This prejudice operates so strongly as almost always to prevent them from ever calling in the same physician again. One physician who had practised with reputation in Marseilles for twenty years, informed me that he was now called in to one family only where he ever had lost a patient. The consequence of this is, that a physician will scarcely venture to order a patient to be bled in a fever, without calling a consultation, to remove the odium that would certainly attach to him (without this precaution,) should his patient die.

There is a public Library and Museum here —the latter of little consequence. The Botanic Garden is small.

The country between Marseilles and Toulon, is very mountainous, though intersected with some beautiful and fertile valleys. Toulon, considered in respect of its climate, has all the faults of Marseilles. Behind the town, in a plain sheltered by some high mountains, the olive-tree attains a size not to be seen about Marseilles. There is, also, a very good Botanic Garden here, and Lectures are given every spring.

HIERES.

About twelve miles beyond Toulon, is situated the small Town of Hieres, much talked of as a winter-residence for consumptive patients. It is said to be completely sheltered from the mistral, which we have seen to be so severely felt at Marseilles; and to possess a mildness —a softness—of climate not to be met with in any other part of Provence. How far it is deserving of this character we shall presently examine. The richness of the country, the beauty of the surrounding hills, clothed almost to the summit with evergreens, and the orange gardens in full bearing, were agreeable objects, which had not greeted our eyes in any other part of Provence : yet, with all these before us, we entered Hieres under the influence of a strong mistral. This was not indeed so bad as I had experienced at Marseilles ; yet it was more than sufficient to convince us, that the high character we had heard of this place, was much overrated.

Hieres is a small ill-built town, prettily
situated on the southern declivity of a hill,
opposite the Islands of the same name, and
about two miles from the shores of the
Mediterranean. The ground between the town
and the sea to the south-east,—with the exception of a small space immediately under the
shelter of the town occupied with orange gardens,—is mostly marshy, and not unfrequently
gives rise to remitting fevers among the inhabitants during the summer. On the north, the
town is well protected by the hills which rise
behind it. To the east and west, there is a large
open valley leaving it exposed to the winds from
those quarters, and even to the north-west.

The country around is very beautiful. The
low grounds are mostly occupied with vines
and corn, and, about the bases of the hills, the
olive attains a large size, and is much cultivated,
—a great part of the riches of the inhabitants
being derived from it. The hills are covered
with a variety of evergreen-shrubs, and the
air perfumed by the wild thyme, rosemary,
lavender, and many other aromatic plants,
several of which I found blooming in December.
So superior, indeed, to any thing we had yet
seen in the south of France, was the whole scene

before us, and so well calculated to convey an impression of great mildness of climate, that, but for the admonitions of the attendant mistral, we should have been led to form high expectations of the amenity of our new residence. This wind we soon found to be of frequent occurrence at Hieres.*

It is true, that about the bases of the hills, there are some spots sheltered from the blasts of the mistral, where the invalid might enjoy several hours in the open air almost every dry day ; but the difficulty is to reach them at the time that they would be most useful. The chilly blast, sweeping round every exposed corner, forbids the valetudinarian venturing there, except in a close carriage ; while, on the other hand, the roads leading to these places do not admit wheeled carriages. The mule with its panniers forms the only means of transport in this neighbourhood, and by these the various offices of husbandry are performed

* The author of a paper on the influence of climate on consumption, in the third No. of the quarterly journal of Foreign Medicine and Surgery, has made a mistake in calling the north-east wind the Mistral. The north-west is the dreaded Mistral of Provence, and most generally brings clear weather with it, whereas easterly winds are generally attended with a damp cloudy atmosphere.

that in most other places are done by carts or waggons.

On referring to the journal of my residence in Hieres, I find that from the 8th, to the 31st, of December, inclusive, there were four whole days of continued rain and three days of partial rain ; two chilly overcast days, with a north-easterly wind ; and nine days during which the wind was steadily at the north-west, accompanied with a clear dry atmosphere. The medium temperature in the shade at 2 P. M. during this time was 50°. A few hours on the 26th, when the weather was calm, was the only time during the above period, on which that class of consumptive invalids generally sent abroad could have been out with advantage, or, I may even say, with safety.

During the first seven days of January, the weather was overcast, damp, and chilly, accompanied with an easterly wind : from the 17th, to the 23rd, it was clear, mild, and pleasant, from there being little wind. The medium temperature in the shade at 2 P. M. was 53°. During this month, there were altogether 18 days in which the invalid might have enjoyed several hours exercise in the middle of the day.

During the last days of this month, and the beginning of February, the weather was cold and stormy. For the two next months of February and March, I subjoin the meteorological tables kept by my friend Mr. Gamble, Surgeon, Royal Navy, who was kind enough to send me a copy of them.*

My endeavours to procure meteorological tables for Hieres for any length of time were fruitless; but I regretted this the less, as, though always deserving attention, the indications of the thermometer, as I have before observed, afford a very inaccurate criterion of the nature of a climate like that of which we are now speaking, so liable to high winds, which affect the living body in a ten fold proportion to what they do the thermometer: And he who, judging simply from the latitude of this country and the tables of the thermometer, shall come to it in hopes of finding the mild weather of his own summer which he has just left behind him, will be woefully disappointed.

A single season is by far too short a period to enable one to form an accurate opinion as to the temperature of any climate or situation,

* See Appendix.

and I was told that the one I had witnessed in
this place, was rather an unfavourable specimen.* Of the situation and exposure of Hieres,
however, my residence was long enough to
enable me to speak with certainty. It is not
well sheltered from the north-east, and still less
so from the north-west, which last we have
noticed as blowing during the greater part of
december, so as to render it unsafe for a consumptive patient to venture out of doors, except
in some corner, where he is exposed to the sun's
rays, and completely sheltered from it.

If any of our medical observations are to be
relied on, the prevalence of a wind like this
must render any situation exposed to its influence
something more than a doubtful one for the
patient labouring under pulmonary cousump-
tion.   The climate of Hieres is more humid
than that of Marseilles.

Though Hieres is not the situation I should
select for a consumptive patient, I have no
hesitation in giving it a decided preference to

---

* I was informed the quantity of rain which fell this season at
Hieres, was greater than usual, whereas at Nice, the quantity I
believe was rather under the average. The comparison drawn
between these two climates from observations made during this
season is therefore fallacious, though I have no doubt but the
climate of Hieres is more humid than that of Nice.

Marseilles. Its exposure is better, and it is in some degree protected by its finely clothed hills from the northerly winds, which, if not warded off, are at least broken in their violence.

The country around this place is open and fine, and the invalid, when the weather does permit him to leave his rooms, may enjoy the advantage of a variety of rides through a beautiful valley, or along the sides of the mountains through paths which present many charming views to amuse the mind, while he enjoys at the same time, the perfume of numerous beautiful and aromatic plants.

Pulmonary consumption, I was informed by the medical men of the place, is far from being a frequent disease at Hieres,—a circumstance which they do not fail to boast of, as well as of the generally healthy state of the climate. Their immunity from consumption (if true) may, perhaps, in some measure, be accounted for by the greater part of the inhabitants of the town, and surrounding district, being much occupied in the labours of the field. The principal source of the wealth of the natives, is derived from the vine and olive, both of which require much labour, particularly the former; and

indeed the greater part of the soil is cultivated
by manual labour.

A few cases of serophula affecting the glands
came under my observation.

The medical practice in the few cases
wherein I witnessed it, was sufficiently inert to
satisfy the warmest advocate of the ' Expectant'
system. In a poor girl, who had been labouring
for weeks under continued fever, with a yellow
skin, frequent bilious vomitings, and a constipated state of the bowels, the Physician expressed surprise at a few grains of calomel being
recommended. It was given, however ; and
its effects, I think, might have convinced the
sturdiest advocate for the *Ptisane System* that
calomel may be useful in some cases. It was
more than sufficient to satisfy the poor patient,
(who, when the load that oppressed her was
removed, had a rapid convalescence,) that she
owed her recovery to it.

The accommodations for invalids at Hieres,
are not very numerous nor comfortable.

I shall now take my leave of this place,
hoping that I have at least given sufficient
information to enable the medical man to form
a tolerably accurate idea of its situation and
climate What I have said of the effect of the

wind here, is still more strongly applicable to
all the other situations in Provence that have
been hitherto recommended as winter residences
for consumptive invalids.

NICE.

NICE with its surrounding valley contains
about 20,000 inhabitants ; and, until the junc-
tion of Genoa to Sardinia, was the principal continental sea-port of that kingdom.   It is built
close to the sea-beach, on a fine bay of the
Mediterranean, about four miles beyond the
river Var, which divides France from the
Sardinian territory.   Behind, and to the westward of the town, extends the beautiful valley
of Nice ;—the last ranges of the Maritime Alps
appearing to retire, and forming a barrier as if
to guard this favoured spot from the influence
of those northern blasts which are so severely
felt in the south of France, for many months
of the year.   From among these mountains,
descends the small river Paglion, scarcely
visible, in general, in its large pebbly bed, the
great extent of which, however, shows its occasional magnitude and force.   This stream
washes the western extremity of the town, and
falls into the bay of Nice.

Immediately beyond this river, and stretch-
ing along the sea-beach for nearly a mile, com-
mences the suburbs of the 'Croix de Marbre',

not unfrequently called the ' Faux-bourg des
Anglois ', from its being the favourite residence
of our countrymen who pass the winter at Nice.
At the western extremity of this Faux-bourg,
rises the range of mountains which shelters it
from the north-west. These form a semicircular
sweep from this point, and terminate in Mon-
talbano, a high mountain which projects into
the sea, immediately to the eastward of the
town. The whole range forms a kind of am-
phitheatre, which at once encloses and shelters
Nice and its beautiful valley. The greatest
distance of the base of these mountains from the
sea-beach, is little more than two miles, and the
breadth of the plain is scarcely so much.

The mountains rise pretty rapidly in ranges,
shewing the gradual decay of their vegetable
covering as they ascend. The eye wanders
from the lower range covered with corn and
vines, growing in the greatest luxuriance under
the shade of the olive, the fig, and a variety of
other fruit-trees, to the lofty and rugged peaks
in the distance whose only covering is snow.

From this arrangement of its mountains,
Nice derives the superior mildness of its climate. While open to the genial influence of
the south, its mountain barrier on all other
sides defends it in a great measure, from the

northerly winds, and particularly from the north-west or mistral. It is not altogether so well sheltered from the north, or rather north-east wind, which sweeping down the valley of the Paglion, is not unfrequently felt during the winter and spring months with considerable severity, but in a degree much inferior, both in frequency and force, to that of the mistral in Provence.*

This superiority of the plains of Nice to any part of the south of France,—I had almost said to any part of the north of Italy,—is observable in the luxuriance of its vegetable productions. I may take the olive and orange-tree as examples of this. At Marseilles, the olive is but a small puny tree, and the orange does not live in the open air during the winter. In the more shel-tered environs of Hieres, the olive-trees are of considerable size, and growing in great abun-dance ; and in the gardens immediately shel-tered by the town and high walls (above which, the branches no sooner raise their heads than they are blasted by their enemy the mistral,)

* Dr. Smollet speaking of the superior mildness of Nice compared to Provence, says " the north and north-west winds blow as cold in Provence, as ever I felt them on the mountains of Scotland : whereas Nice is altogether screened from these winds by the Mari-time Alps." Travels—Letter 24th.

the orange-tree thrives and produces abundance
of fruit. It is of that species, however, which
is least sensible to cold. At Nice we find the
olive has attained the full size. It is here a
lofty tree, throwing forth its branches with a
luxuriance, and exhibiting a richness of foliage
not to be met with in France, and producing a
proportionate quantity of fruit; while the orange,
in almost all its varieties, grows in abundance
in the plains, with comparatively little regard
to shelter from walls, depending chiefly on its
great alpine barriers for protection. We might
shew the superior warmth of Nice further, by
pointing out several productions of the vegetable kingdom which thrive in it, and are unknown in the other places alluded to ; but the
instance we have adduced is probably sufficient.

Nothing can exceed the high state of cul-
tivation of the country about Nice. The whole
is like a garden. Wherever there is a particle
of soil along the ridges of the mountains it is
turned to use. If corn will not grow the vine
or the olive often will, even when the depth of
the soil is almost nothing. All is performed by
manual labour.

" L'industrie des habitans de cette contrée,"
says a native author, " a convertie en bosquets
d'oliviers et de caroubiers les collines et les
falaises steriles de la côte, et couverte la base
de ces élévations de jardins magnifiques où
l'oranger, le bigarradier, le limettier, le cèdra-
tier, et le limonier ou citronnier, étalent une
verdure perpetuelle, exhalent un parfum deli-
cieux, et donnent des fruits excellens."*

After all this industry the country is still incapable of maintaining its inhabitants, and they
accordingly receive supplies from the more fertile plains of Piedmont on the other side of the
Maritime Alps.

The increased vigour and more advanced
progress of vegetation on our way from Hieres
to Nice, we first observed immediately after
crossing the Estrelles, a range of high mountains between Hieres and Antibes which appear

---

* Essai sur L'Histoire des Orangers par M. Risso. I take this
opportunity of acknowledging my obligations to this gentleman for
much information, and also for the meteorological tables for Nice,
which were kept by him with great accuracy, and which will be found
in the Appendix. Besides the work just quoted, M. R. is author of
a work on the Natural History of the *Fishes* of the Mediterranean, and
also of several other works. The cultivator of Natural History who
visits Nice, will find in M. R. a valuable acquaintance.

to form the first barrier to the progress of the mistral.

The most sheltered part of the valley of Nice is that lying behind the Croix de Marbre; and there, a little way on the northern side of the road, among the orange gardens, or about the base of the hills, will be found the most favourable residence for the invalid. This spot is far preferable to the best situation in the town, where it is impossible to avoid exposure to currents of air in traversing the streets, which, however, must be done, if the invalid wishes to enjoy the advantages of a country ride. The wind is, besides, often felt much more in the town than in many parts of the country, as I have had frequent opportunities of observing.

Often have I left the town when the wind was blowing with considerable violence, and, on visiting some of my friends in the situations mentioned, I have found them so well sheltered, that, but for the waving of the olive trees on the surrounding hills, or the rapid motion of the clouds, we should not have known that there was any wind. This is strikingly evinced by an observation in an excellent paper on the climate of Nice, published in Dr. Thomson's Annals for September, 1818. " And even in

the neighbourhood of Nice, it might in the same
manner be observed, that some situations were
much more eligible than others in point of
shelter and warmth, though not so evident at
first sight. After a visit by a very cold, bleak,
and violent mistral in the month called April,
its mischievous effects were very observable
upon the tender vine shoots as well as upon the
young green leaves of the mulberry trees, in
shrivelling them as if they had been burned,
leaving but a poor prospect for the next vintage,
and throwing back considerably the ensuing
crop of silk. I observed these effects particularly between Antibes and the valley of the
Var; also in many situations in the valleys
about Nice, which ran north and south; but in
other places on the south sides of the hills, the
mulberry trees mostly escaped uninjured, and
in some instances were to be seen in a flourish-
ing state, at a little distance from others which
were blasted, but which had not been so protected."

The soil about Nice is remarkably dry, yet
there is no deficiency of water, as several large
sources issue from the base of the surrounding
mountains, and traverse the valley in their progress to the sea. This water is generally hard,
owing to the neighbouring hills being chiefly
composed of calcareous rocks.

Provisions are good and abundant at Nice, and the same may be said of the domestic accommodations, making allowance always for the inconveniences, which, to an English family, are inseparable from all foreign houses.

The great fault of all the houses in these climates is their being built with too little regard to the short period in which cold weather prevails. The proportion of this to the warm is so little, that it seems to be lost sight of altogether in planning the houses.

The *Climate* of Nice, speaking generally, is dry, though not so much so as that of Marseilles. It is considered very steady during the winter, and I believe is as much so as most places on the continent. It is still more remarkable for the beauty and brilliancy of its skies. This is well remarked and illustrated by the author of the paper on the climate of Nice, already quoted. " The clearness of the atmosphere, (he says) was very remarkable ; the moon and the stars appeared very brilliant, and the lofty mountains of Corsica, with their snowy summits, were occasionally to be seen by the naked eye, rising above the south-eastern horizon, at a direct distance of about 120, or 130 miles (English)". The quantity of rain which falls in different seasons varies very considerably. I may remark here, that there must, I think, have been some error in the Thermometer used by Dr. Smollet, or in his manner of taking his observations, as his tables are at such variance with all others that I have seen. Such a change of climate as his tables indicate, can scarcely have taken place in the space of less than sixty years. The quantity of rain, too, that fell during the second winter of Dr. Smollett's residence, is very remarkable, particularly when contrasted with that of 1817, and 1818. From the middle of November, to 20th of March, during the former, there were 56 days of rain, while during the whole of the six winter months, in the latter, there were only 25; and even this, it appears from the tables in the appendix, is a proportion considerably beyond the mean.*

Nice is protected from the dreaded mistral but is still subject to some winds chiefly the north-east, east, and south-east, which, though they do not blow with the violence of those of Provence, nevertheless are sharp and cold. They are particularly frequent during the spring months, and form a strong objection, in my opinion, to the climate as a spring residence for

* See Appendix.

the consumptive. During the existence of
these keen winds, the difference of temperature
between the sun and the shade, is very considerable, and cannot fail to be injurious to such invalids. The liability of Nice to these spring
winds constitutes an essential part of the character of its climate. They were very frequent
in the spring of 1818, and I found them much
complained of by strangers, even those in health.
To those who had passed the whole season
there, the change between the spring and winter
months, (which latter are comparatively little
liable to those winds,) appeared very remarkable.

Dr. Smollet who passed two winters at Nice,
and who was the first, I believe, who brought
it into notice as a winter's residence, particularly
remarks this change between the winter and
spring. After a few observations on the dryness of the climate, he says: " In a word, I
passed the winter here, much more comfortably
than I expected.—About the vernal equinox,
however, I caught a violent cold, which was
attended with a difficulty of breathing ; and
as the sun advances towards the tropic, I find
myself still more subject to rheunis. As
the heat increases, the humours of the body
are rarified, and of consequence the pores of
the skin are opened ; while the east-wind

sweeping over the Alps and Appenines, covered with snow, continues surprizingly *sharp* and *penetrating.* Even the people of the country who enjoy good health, are afraid of exposing themselves to the air at this season, the intemperature of which may last till the middle of May."* " In March and April", he observes in another place, " I would not advise a valetudinarian to go forth without taking precautions against the cold." Again, after relating the good effects of the climate on some nervous patients, he says : " In winter, but especially in the spring, the sun is so hot, that one can hardly take exercise of any sort abroad, without being thrown into a breathing sweat; and the wind, at this season, is so cold and piercing, that it often produces a mischievous effect on the pores thus opened ; the people are then subject to colds, pleurisies, peripneumonies, and ardent fevers."† Dr. Smollet's observations on this occasion deserve the more attention, as he was himself a valetudinarian. During the prevalence of these winds in 1818, several of the consumptive patients were attacked by Hæmoptysis. The medical men of Nice, whom I generally found disposed to speak well of their

---

* Travels in France and Italy.—Letter 37.

† Ib. ....—Letter 24.

climate as a residence for consumptive patients
during the months of November, December,
and January, themselves allowed that the frequent occurrence of the keen winds of the three
following months, rendered it an unfavourable
one during that time.

Now, allowing that the climate during the
winter months is favourable in cases of pulmonary consumption,—a circumstance, which we
shall presently enquire into,—the invalid who
winters there, must submit also to remain during the spring months, as he can only venture
to leave the place by sea, in order to change his
present for a better situation, and the opportunities for doing this with any comfort are very rare.
This is no small objection to Nice ; as, however
medical men may differ about the effects of the
winter months on consumptive invalids, there
can be but one opinion, I think, after what has
been stated, of it as a spring climate. The invalid who goes to spend the winter there, and
has objections to a sea voyage, or cannot procure a comfortable vessel, must not venture to
leave it till the month of May, by any of the
usual roads.

Two families in April, 1818, did so by crossing the ' Col de Tende', a high mountain, over
which the road from Nice to Turin passes.

Both suffered from the effects of the cold, and particularly one Lady who was obliged to be carried over the snow in a chair. This passage ought not to be attempted by the invalid before May, and I am acquainted with a family who were detained at the foot of this mountain, by a snow-storm even in the beginning of that month. On the other hand, if the stranger returns by France, he has to cross the Estrelles, and will, besides, on entering Provence, find a great difference between its climate, and that of the sheltered valley he has left, Two invalids that did so, and went to Aix in April, suffered not a little from their imprudence.

The following information relating to the diseases of the Nizards, I obtained from the medical men of the place.

The Inhabitants of Nice may be considered as generally healthy. Their most frequent diseases are Catarrhal affections. Pulmonary consumption, without being very frequent, carries off many of the inhabitants annually, occurring more frequently in the town than in the country. Of four hundred patients in the practice of Dr. Perez, a respectable physician, in 1817, there were sixteen of pulmonary consumption. Of these eleven died. Tubercles, he gave as the most frequent cause of the disease, and

in some cases neglected catarrh.* Cutaneous
diseases are common. Epidemic fevers, said to
be of the typhoid or putrid character, occur,
but at long intervals. Cancerous affections are
not unfrequent. Rheumatism is not common ;
indeed it is one of the diseases in which this
climate is said to be particularly useful. I met
with a striking example of this in a German
gentleman, whose rheumatism did not trouble
him at Nice, though he had been subject to it
every winter for many years in other places.
Gout is another disease in which the climate is
said to be useful. The other diseases which are
said to derive benefit from a residence here are
the indefinite class of nervous affections ; Dys-
pepsia; Hypochondriasis, &c. And these are

* The general belief of the inhabitants is, that this disease (Consumption) has only appeared among them since strangers have come
to pass the winter at Nice. They believe that it is infectious, and
change or destroy the furniture of a room in which such patients die.

This is a very prevalent belief in the southern parts of Europe. At
Rome a gentleman of my acquaintance was refused lodgings from a
suspicion that he was consumptive; and it was only after a friend's
engaging to pay for all the furniture of the lodgings, should he die,
that he was admitted. It is not long since a law existed in Rome, by
which the proprietor of the house wherein a consumptive patient
died, could claim payment of his furniture which was burnt. Some
other cases similar to the above have come to my knowledge, and
should render the friends of consumptive patients cautious in mentioning the nature of their complaints.

the diseases which, from the nature of the
climate, we should expect to be benefited by it.
Scrophula is rarely met with—Calculus vesicæ is
also rare.

The general Hospital is sufficiently large to
contain about a hundred patients, and is kept
in tolerably good order. The cases during my
residence there were mostly chronic. The medical practice, from the few opportunities I had
of observing it, appeared to differ little from
what I have already remarked in the south of
France. I found here the same fondness for
consultations ;—a practice, the great prevalence
of which shows either a want of confidence on
the part of the community in their medical men,
or a timidity and indecision on the part of the
latter to put in practice what their own knowledge suggests to them as best.

One of the features in the practice of medicine in France, by which it strikingly differs
from that in England, is, the frequency of these
consultations, and the number of medical men
assembled at them : were I to form an opinion
from the result of not a few of these, I should
say it formed one of the *faults* as well as features
of the French practice.

Having now given some idea of the local situation of Nice, of the general nature of its climate, and of the advantages in this respect which it possesses over the south of France; and having, also, given the little information relative to the diseases of the inhabitants which I obtained from the resident medical men ; I come to consider the subject to which all these observations lead : viz. What are the effects of the climate of Nice upon patients labouring under pulmonary consumption? Is the practice of sending such patients from England to pass the winter in this place, founded on certain experience of its utility ? or is it not rather, taking into consideration the disadvantages of so long a journey, in many cases injurious ?

These are grave and important questions; and if it should appear to be the result of our enquiries that more injury, upon the whole, than benefit, may be expected from the practice of sending consumptive invalids to Nice, (especially after the disease has made some progress,) it cannot fail to excite surprize that this practice has continued so long, more especially when we consider the great number of medical men (many of these having the particular charge of consumptive patients) that have visited Nice since Dr. Smollet brought it into note sixty years ago.

And yet, when we consider that the now neglected Montpelier was once as famous as even Nice was some years since, and as it still continues to be in the estimation of many English physicians, the most unfavourable issue to our investigation ought, perhaps, to create less wonder than we might, on the first view, be led to entertain. For my own part I have no hesitation in expressing my belief, that, before very many years, the English physician will no more think of sending his consumptive patients to the latter place than to the former.

In thus strongly stating my opinion on this point, I beg it to be understood that it is not founded solely on the limited experience which my short stay at Nice permitted me to acquire ; although, doubtlessly, without my own personal observation, information drawn from other sources would have had less weight. When, however, the observations and opinions derived from various and respectable quarters mutually corroborate one another, and strikingly harmonize with mine, I confess I feel much less hesitation in expressing my own sentiments on the important subject in question.

Were I to take the melancholy progress of
consumption among those of my countrymen
whom I met at Nice, as affording sufficient
data to form an opinion as to the effects of its
climate in this disease, I should, indeed, have
little hesitation in making up my mind; but I
know too well the fatal career of this disease in
a very large proportion of cases in every climate,
and in every variety of circumstances, to judge
from an experience so limited as this, however
striking and uniform.

This is a point, on which, as I have already
said, the united experience of many only can
decide ; and it is much to be regretted, that so
few of the medical men who have visited this
place, have given us their opinion of it.   It is a
duty which they who have an opportunity of visiting these climates owe to their countrymen,
to communicate the observations they make,
however few, in order that their medical brethren at home, who have not had the same advantage, may be enabled to form an opinion on
a matter of such vital interest to society at large.

The generality of authors, it is true, who
have mentioned Nice, have, like myself, resided
there for too short a period to entitle their
opinions to very much weight ; but no one, as
far as I know, has given his opinion in *favour*

of it as a climate in pulmonary consumption ;
at least, where that opinion was founded on actual observation.   Indeed, the information to be
found in medical, or other authors on this point,
is very unsatisfactory ; no greater proof of which
need be mentioned than the uncertainty respecting our present enquiries which exists among
medical men in general.

Amidst this difference of sentiment, I have
much satisfaction in being able to state the
opinion of a physician, whose opportunities of
observation have, I presume, been more extensive than those of any medical writer who
has treated of Nice; so extensive, indeed, as
to render his opinions obnoxious to none of
the objections to which my own observations,
and those of other writers already alluded to
are liable.   The person I allude to, is Professor
FODERE of Strasbourg, the author of the most
learned and useful work on medical jurisprudence that has appeared, and of several other
much esteemed productions.   During a residence of upwards of six years at that place,
Dr. Fodere was particularly occupied in attending to the natural history of the country, and
the effects of the climate on disease.

In conversation with this eminent physician
in July last, I took an opportunity of stating to

him the strong doubts that I entertained on the
propriety of sending our consumptive patients
to Nice. On this occasion, he not only stated
very fully to me his own opinions, but kindly
permitted me to extract his matured observations from a large work which he has had ready
for the press, for some time past, on the natural
history, &c. of the Maritime Alps—a work containing much interesting and valuable information. In a conversation with him at another
time, about some points of little consequence,
in which our observations were a little at variance, he concluded by the following remark:
—" There is one thing certain, Sir, you may
safely assure your countrymen, that it is a very
bad practice to send their consumptive patients
to die at Nice".

What weight Professor Foderé's opinions
and observations may have in deciding the judgment of other medical men upon the effects of
the climate of this place, I know not, but I
confess, when added to the observations I had
an opportunity of making myself, they leave
very little doubt on my mind of its being, at
least, *useless* in *any* stage of the complaint, and
worse than useless in the latter stage of pulmonary consumption.

1 translate the extracts from Professor
Foderé's work literally.

" I come at length, (he says) to that terrible disease which carries off, annually, the
tenth part of the inhabitants of Europe and
North-America—*pulmonary consumption.* Since
we have shown that scrophulous affections are
by no means rare among the Maritime Alps, it
will naturally be expected that this other malady
is also found ; and, accordingly, I have to remark, that pectoral affections are common at
Nice, Villa Franca, and along the whole coast
where scrophula prevails. I have always been
astonished that our older physicians should
have sent their consumptive patients to our sea
shores ; since it seems irrefragably proved by
the experience of our time, that the climate of
the shores of the Mediterranean is hurtful to
such invalids. 1 had seen a great number of
these cases terminate fatally at Marseilles, and,
at that time, I considered the very dry and keen
winds of that place, as the principal source of
evil ; but I afterwards found that the warmer,
softer, and more humid atmosphere of Nice, was
in no respect more favourable to such complaints.   Every case of hereditary tubercular
phthisis proves fatal, as well at Nice as at Villa
Franc, in very early age.   In these places

consumption is not, as in Switzerland, on the
Banks of the Soane, and in Alsace, a chronic
disease: on the contrary, I have very often seen
it terminate in forty days. A physician of the
countries just mentioned would be surprized
at the quickness with which one attack of
Hæmoptysis succeeds another, how readily the
tubercles suppurate, and how speedily the lungs
are destroyed. The English annually make
fresh experience of this melancholy fact, and
their burying ground in the *Croix de Marbre*
too well testifies its truth.

" In considering what may be the causes of
this uncommon frequency and fatality of consumption in this country, many are disposed to
lay much stress on the sudden variations of its
climate. But, let me ask, in what countries
are not such variations found? And in what
book of medicine are they not accused as the
manifold source of diseases? And yet the rapid
career of consumption, which we have just
noticed, is very uncommon in most other countries, even in such as are cold and moist. In
these, the disease, although without offering
any solid hopes of a cure, gives, nevertheless,
a long truce to its victims. From this it would
appear that there must be on the shores of the
Mediterranean some other source of evil beside

mere variability of climate; and I am disposed
to look for this in the impregnation of its atmosphere with some of the muriatic salts of the
neighbouring ocean.

" Upon the whole I consider it as contrary
to observation and experience, to send patients
affected with tubercular Phthisis to the sea
coast. And yet it is singular that the practice
should continue to be persisted in. If ever a
cure of the disease has been obtained by such a
measure, of which I much doubt, it must, I
conceive, have been in cases of spurious or
mucous consumptions only." In another place
Professor Foderé has the following remark:
" I have observed that there is a tendency in
the diseases of these places to attack the organs
of respiration; and this is proved, independently
of the symptoms during life, by examinations
after death, which prove the lungs to be much
more frequently gorged with blood and in-
durated (hepatisés) than in other countries."

He observes, also, that persons predisposed
to phthisical complaints do not die in summer,
but in the autumn, when the mornings and evenings begin to get cold, and augment the conges-
tion of the lungs by checking the perspiration.

For many other valuable remarks on this and other subjects I could refer the reader to this work of the learned Professor, if, indeed, its publication rendered it accessible.*

As strikingly corroborative of the fact detailed by Professor Foderé of the uncommon prevalence and fatality of consumptive diseases on the shores of the Mediterranean, I am enabled to give the reader some extracts from another document, which, although published, is, perhaps, nearly equally inaccessible as the professor's. The work to which I allude is a Thesis published at Edinburgh in 1817,† by Dr. Samuel Sinclair, Surgeon in the Royal Navy. In the beginning of his essay, Dr. S. informs us that the observations contained in it are the result of several years' service in the Mediterranean, and especially in the fleet employed off the southern shores of France. Speaking of the practice of sending consumptive

* Histoire Naturelle, Agraire et Medicale du Comté de Nice et pays limitrophes. M. S.

† *De impulsu quo cœlum maris mediterranei pulmones afficit.* My attention was first called to this little work by a short notice of it in the last edition of the invaluable work on tropical climates by my friend Dr. Johnson.

patients to the South of France, he says, " I
am the more desirous of making known the
results of my own experience in this matter, as
I am well convinced that the prevalent opinions
respecting it are most erroneous. So far from
coinciding with these opinions, I must declare,
that I am borne out by the united experience of
all my medical friends, who have served in that
country, in asserting, that the climate of the
Mediterranean, more especially at certain seasons of the year, is particularly hostile to, and
productive of, pulmonary complaints!"

These are strong assertions, but they seem
borne out, as far at least as *seamen* are concerned, by the official statements adduced by
Dr. S. in support of his opinions. From these
it appears, that during the years 1810, 1811,
and 1812, there were admitted into the naval
hospitals of the Mediterranean, from the fleet,
(which contained about thirty thousand men,)
four hundred and fifty-five cases of Phthisis
Pulmonalis, and one hundred and forty of Pneumonia,—making a proportion of one in sixty-
five affected with the former complaint, or of
one in fifty when the two diseases are taken
together.* This proportion of pulmonic disease

* See Appendix.

is certainly very great; much greater, no doubt,
than is observed among the same class of persons, and under similar circumstances, in most
other parts of the world. On this account, I
think we must admit Dr. Sinclair's evidence
as strong against the idea of the beneficial influence of the shores of the Mediterranean in
complaints of the lungs. It is, however, not
to be overlooked that the cases of seamen
navigating the Mediterranean seas, and of
persons residing at their ease on its shores,
are very dissimilar. In the case of the seaman
there are many causes tending directly to
affect the pulmonary system, from which the
resident on shore is exempt. Of these Dr. S.
enumerates frequent alternations of temperature
in the performance of his duties,—sleeping on
the decks at night,—abuse of spirituous liquors,
&c. And we also find this author, in opposition to some other writers, stating consumption
to be a frequent disease among seamen in
general. Dr. S. is, however, decidedly of
opinion, also, that the prevalence of consumptive diseases is infinitely greater among this class
of men in the Mediterranean, than on the shores
of the north of Europe. He adduces an interesting fact in proof of the evil influence of the
Mediterranean climate on the lungs, from his

own experience, which I shall quote:—" In the severe winter of 1814 the Colossus ship of the line, of which I was then surgeon, remained the greater part of the season in the river Scheldt, inclosed in the ice. During this time Faren-heit's thermometer continued much below the freezing point,—for several weeks as low even as 18°; yet, on this occasion, the number of men attacked with catarrh and pneumonia was seldom so great as I had witnessed, during the preceding *summer* and *autumn*, in the *Medi-terranean*, among a crew of only one half the number (three hundred). Acute Rheumatism, however, a disease of rare occurrence in the Mediterranean, was here very prevalent. I need hardly mention, as explanatory of these different results, that the temperature though low, was very uniform in the former instance."*

As accounting for this extraordinary preva-lence of pulmonary disease in the Mediterranean, Dr. S. enumerates the following causes :—First and principally, the peculiar nature of the *cli-mate*, which he describes as being singularly variable and uncertain. Speaking of this he says—" It is indeed true, that it may claim anim-

* P. 17.

munity from the great permanent heat of the tropical, and cold of the northern regions ; but it is subject to an inconstancy of weather, and an irregularity of temperature altogether unknown in either of these".* The climate acts secondarily, also, by exciting diseases (the principal of which is fever) that leave a predisposition to pulmonic affections. Dr. S. enumerates, in the third place, the peculiar duties and habits and mode of life of seamen, as partly accounting for the uncommon frequency of the disease in their particular case.

The disease, as described by this author, appears to belong to that species termed Apostematous by Dr. Duncan ; and on this account also, his observations are perhaps not so applicable to the hereditary tubercular Phthisis which constitutes the great majority of cases that are sent abroad for relief. It appears to have been uncommonly rapid, and to equal, in this respect, the complaint as described by Foderé at Nice, and Dr. Segaud, at Marseilles. It proved sometimes fatal in a few weeks, and was rarely protracted beyond five or six months. He has seen the lungs almost entirely consumed in the space of six weeks from the first attack of inflammation.

* P. 9.

In his section on the cure of this disease, **Dr.
S.** strongly urges the propriety of a speedy return
to England. So universally experienced, indeed,
was the rapidity and untractable nature of this
disease in the Mediterranean, that the comman-
der in chief issued an order, that those attacked
by it should be permitted to return to England
by the first opportunity, without waiting for the
formal process of being invalided : a practice,
the propriety of which appears to be well justified by the fact, stated by Dr. S., that many
thus sent home recovered.*

* As bearing upon the opinion maintained by Professor Fodéré, and
some other writers, respecting the evil influence of marine exhalations
in exciting consumptive diseases, the facts brought forward by Dr.
Sinclair, may probably be claimed by the advocates of each doctrine,
as supporting their own side of the question. For my own part,
although from several circumstances that have come to my knowledge,
(some of which are alluded to in this work) rather inclined to the opinion of the hostile influence of a marine atmosphere, I am obliged to
confess, after an impartial review of Dr. Sinclair's essay, that the
facts contained in it seem very conclusive on the other side. These
facts and the arguments founded on them, that lead to this conclusion,
may be shortly stated thus : Consumption is a frequent disease among
seamen in general ; it is much more frequent among them in the
Mediterranean than on other stations : Its frequency among seamen in
general, (even admitting it to be more frequent than among persons
in civil life, which is not asserted,) is not by any means greater than
can be well accounted for by several circumstances in their peculiar
mode of life (exclusive of the mere fact of their living on the ocean)
enumerated by Dr. S. and others ; the increased proportion, then, in
the Mediterranean must be owing to other and more local causes than
the simple impregnation of its atmosphere with some of the saline
contents of the sea.

With these observations I shall take my
leave of the climate of Nice. Any invalid
wishing to try the effects of a winter there, should
endeavour to get to it towards the end of October,
or early in November, and remain till the beginning of May. Whatever inconveniences he may
suffer from the spring winds, he would probably
suffer still more in attempting, as some do, to cross
the mountains to the north of Italy, or in returning by the Estrelles to the south of France.

It is true, the invalid, if he can bear the fa-
tigue of riding on a mule, may leave Nice
much sooner for Italy by the coast road. On
this route, he has nothing to dread from a
change of climate, as the road leads the whole
way along the sea-shore, at the foot of high
mountains, through many fine valleys.

The journey performed in this way to Genoa
will ocupy four or five days. The accommodations on this road are however not the best suited
for an invalid.

It was by this route that Napoleon intended
to carry the excellent road that was to join the
south of France with Italy, and which is made
as far as Menton, sixteen miles beyond Nice.
At this little town we were struck with the
different looks of the people, particularly the
women, whose fine complexions formed a

striking contrast with the generally sallow
countenances of the inhabitants about Nice.
What could be the cause of this striking difference of complexion in climates and situations so
similar? The sheltered little valley of Menton
is almost filled with Lemon-trees, which require
a warmer climate than the orange. They form
the chief article of culture here. This beautiful
ever-green,—which we found still covered with
blossoms and fruit, in the various stages, from
the first formation to maturity,—is far more
prolific than the orange, which merely produces one crop annually. A thousand oranges
are considered a good return for a full grown
orange-tree, while a lemon-tree has been known
to produce eight thousand lemons in one year.

While on the subject of travelling in this part
of the country, I must caution the invalid
against the common practice of descending the
Rhone from Lyons to Avignon, which is far
from being a safe measure. The valley of the
Rhone is often very narrow, the mountains on
each side encroaching closely on the banks of
the river. This conformation of the locality
produces frequent high winds, which are often
severely felt by the invalid. In addition, the
passengers, on the occurrence of bad weather,

are often obliged to stop at places where the accommodations are very bad. One gentleman who had passed the summer well in England, and whom I met with in this very predicament, told me some months after, on seeing me at Nice, that he had not then got the better of the cold he had caught on the Rhone.

VILLA FRANCA.

The author of a paper in a late Number of
the Quarterly Journal of Foreign Medicine and
Surgery, has spoken in very high terms of the
warm sheltered situation of Villa Franca. That
it is more sheltered from northerly winds than
Nice is certain ; and that it possesses a higher
temperature I also believe ; yet I was rather
surprized to find that the difference of the average monthly minimum temperature amounted
to six degrees in favour of Villa Franca. This
place is separated from Nice only by Montal-
bano, which forms the western side of a beautiful
and spacious harbour, at the bottom of which it
lies. It is sheltered effectually from all northerly
winds, by the range of lofty mountains at the base
of which it is built. It is a small insignificant
place. To the eastward of the town and harbour is a small plain, the only level piece of
ground in the neighbourhood. Though sheltered from the north, Villa Franca is open to
the full influence of the east and south-east
winds, which we have noticed as forming an objection to Nice as a spring climate. The cli-

mate of Villa Franca is considerably drier than
that of Nice. Dr. Foderé found a very remarkable difference in this respect in favour of Villa
Franca, by accurate Hygrometric observations.

This quality of dryness, although it may
be of advantage in some diseases, will not
be considered so, I believe, by the generality
of medical men in pulmonary consumption.
This however is another point which still remains
to be settled. The truth I believe is, that no
particular climate will be found to agree with
all cases of this disease ; yet there can be little
doubt that there is one kind of climate which
will be found more generally useful than any
other. Of the advantages of a mild equable
temperature, in pulmonary consumption, there
is little or no difference of opinion ; but medical men are not equally agreed upon the advantages, or disadvantages, to be derived from the
secondary qualities of dryness and moisture.
Speaking of moisture, the learned author of the
' Essay on the medical effects of climates,' observes,—" moisture is supposed, by some, to
be favourable, by others, to be unfavourable,
to such persons (the consumptive) ; it may therefore be safely neglected, except as tending to

increase the evils depending on a want of equability of temperature."*

In this I cannot agree with Dr. Young. I believe the subject of too much importance to be set aside without enquiry, and though it is deviating somewhat from the line I had prescribed to myself in drawing up these observations, I cannot let the present occasion pass without making a few remarks on this subject. The medical men on the continent, as far as I had an opportunity of enquiring, seem agreed on the *superiority* of a moist climate in the generality of cases of pulmonary consumption According to their observation, this quality of climate, even when combined with cold, seems to retard the progress of the disease. Professor Foderé, who has paid much attention to the subject, is decidedly of this opinion. Even in the cold moist climate of Strasbourg, he has found the disease to have much more of a chronic nature than in the territory of Nice ; its average duration, as he informed me, being in the former place about two years.

In the 'Dictionnaire des Sciences Medicales' the advantages of a mild moist atmosphere in this disease, is frequently stated ; among others in the articles *Humidité* and *Hygrométrie*. Dr.

* Treatise on Consumption—.p 85.

Currie found the cold and moist air of Matlock to agree with him. With regard to the moist state of the air caused by the vicinity of the sea, I have already made some remarks.

The effects of this particular kind of moisture, is another point on which medical opinion is at variance, and 1 apprehend that a much greater collection of facts than at present exist, are still wanted finally to decide the matter in question.

But to return to Villa Franca :* This place, I am of opinion, must share the fate of Nice, as to its climate, whatever that may be; for though more sheltered from northerly winds, it has all the other good and bad qualities of the latter

---

* After perusing many excellent remarks in the paper (in the Quarterly Journal) so often above alluded to, I was much disappointed when I came to that part of it which treats of particular climates, to find it so liable to the same objections as were noticed in the beginning of this Essay, as accounting for the uncertainty of medical opinion on this subject : I shall only notice one instance of this. After censuring some authors for condemning particular situations because they were in the vicinity of mountains, &c. without considering other circumstances, we find the writer falling into the very same error, in condemning with one sweep of his pen, Florence, Rome, and Naples, because " the neighbourhood of the Appenines is here the unhappy circumstance"! Assuredly the Author must be totally unacquainted with the situations, respecting which he writes, from personal observation, else he could never have classed together places so very differently circumstanced as these are, in almost every respect of climate and local position.

place, with the additional disadvantage of possessing few or no accommodations for invalids. On these accounts, therefore, notwithstanding the very high encomiums passed upon it by the author alluded to,—encomiums, too, we may remark, as far as regard the effects of the climate, in the disease which is the object of our enquiry, entirely gratuitous,—I am strongly inclined to believe that it will never become the resort of invalids.

―――――

PISA.

PISA is a pretty large well-built town, containing about eighteen thousand inhabitants,
situated on the banks of the Arno, (which runs
through it nearly from east to west,) about six
miles from the sea. The country around it is
flat and moist. To the north of the town lie
some hills which are said to shelter it from the
north wind, but they appear to me too distant
to perform that office well. They certainly do
not protect it from the coldest wind, the north-
east. This opinion was confirmed by the as-
surance of Mr. Zannini, professor of Astronomy
in the University, who stated this to be the
coldest wind. To this gentleman I am indebted
for much attention, and the excellent meteorological tables for Pisa, which will be found in
the appendix.* The same gentleman informed
me that the climate of Pisa is very variable, and
subject to high winds in the autumn, and also,
and more particularly, in the spring. Compared
with the climate of Nice, he informed me, the
average temperature given by the thermometer

* See Appendix.

I

is lower; and on comparing my tables of Nice
with his I found this to be the case. By the
tables given in the appendix it appears that the
mean monthly temperature of Nice, for the six
winter months, is $3\frac{2}{3}°$ higher than that of Pisa.
In the month of February the difference amounts
to 5°· in favour of Nice. The difference of
latitude between Marseilles, Hieres, Nice,
and Pisa is so trifling, as not to be worth remarking, all these places being in the same
degree of latitude, 43°; the mean annual temperature of which, according to professor Leslie's
calculations is 59°.

The northern bank of the Arno, (where the
houses are built in a kind of crescent form, following the sweep of the river, facing the south,
and protected from the north winds,) is generally chosen as the residence of the invalids that
winter at Pisa. In this situation, I was told,
owing to its direct exposure to the sun, the
temperature often rises high, (even during the
prevalence of the sharp cold northerly winds,)
causing a kind of artificial climate, which
requires much care on the part of the invalid,
and which, I apprehend, is of very doubtful
utility. The sharp spring winds which I have
described as being so prevalent at Nice, are also

the worst part of the climate of Pisa.* Pisa is
only six miles distant from the sea, and as the
whole country between it and the shore is a
continued flat, it is of course fully exposed to
the influence of a maritime exposure—whatever
that may be.

Whether Pisa possesses much advantage
over Nice as a residence for consumptive
patients during the six winter months, requires,
I believe, to be proved   We have brought forward pretty strong evidence on the effects to be
expected from the climate of Nice, and I know
of no direct evidence in favour of that of Pisa.
Indeed I am not aware that any medical man
has published any thing on the subject. It is
to be hoped the matter will not be allowed to
rest long in its present state.

To those who come to Italy by sea, Nice
and Pisa are almost similarly circumstanced in
point of convenience, the former being a sea
port, and the latter only sixteen miles distant
from Leghorn. The land journey is certainly
considerably longer to Pisa than to Nice, and to

* I have already mentioned Prof. Zannini's information on this
point; and Dr. Kissock, who called on me while writing these pages,
stated in very strong terms, the sharpness with which he had felt these
winds. Dr. K. had passed the spring of 1818 at Pisa.

some invalids that may be an object. The dangers said to attend crossing the Alps I, however, consider of no moment. They may be crossed with perfect safety, I believe, by any invalid, who should think of a journey to Italy, by Mount Cenis, or the Simplon, at any time between June and October. Pisa possesses one advantage over Nice, namely, that there are good roads leading from it to all parts of Italy, and the invalid may leave it with safety much sooner than he could Nice.

ROME.

The great numbers of our countrymen who annually resort to this wonderful city, and the circumstance of its not unfrequently being preferred as a winter residence by the invalid, will, I hope, render the following observations on its climate, imperfect as they are, acceptable to the medical reader.

During the season the Author passed at Rome, the month of November was fine and mild, with little rain or wind. The first twenty days of December were variable but mild. On the twentieth the weather became colder with a clear atmosphere and sharp northerly wind, (Tramontana), but at the same time very light. This weather continued without varying till the fifteenth of January, when the wind shifted to the westward and southward, and became much milder. During the last days of this month much rain fell. The month of February was very variable and rainy during the last eight days. This was altogether the most unpleasant month we had. In the early part of March we had still some rain, but the greater part of this

month was fair and mild. The northerly or
north-westerly breezes, which occasionally blow
pretty strongly, felt rather cold, but, as far as
I could trust to my own feelings, they were not
to be compared, in frequency or effect, to the
keen chilling winds of Nice at the same season.
The month of April was very fine, and the
weather continued cool and pleasant up to the
10th of May, after which I had no farther opportunity of observing it.

No correct opinion of a climate can be
formed from the observations made during a
single season, and much less when that season
is a very unusual one, as was the case with the
winter of 1818 and 1819 at Rome, when these
observations were made. The long continued
clear weather of December and January, and
the degree of cold accompanying it, are unusual occurrences in that city.*

The climate of Rome differs considerably
from that of Nice and the southern parts of

* Though not inattentive to the state of the thermometer during
my residence at Rome, my observations were not made with that re-
gularity which could enable me to form any accurate conclusions ;
and I have to regret being disappointed in getting some others more to
be depended on, kept by a scientific gentleman of Rome. See Appendix.

Provence. It is more moist. The dry cold winds experienced at these places are comparatively little felt at Rome.

The greater part of the town, built on the Ancient Campus Martius, lies low, and is tolerably well sheltered, by the surrounding rising grounds, from the northerly winds. The seven hills and the Pincian lie between the lower parts of the town and the marshy grounds on the south-east side. Except when it rained, there were few days during this unfavourable winter that the invalid might not have enjoyed a couple of hours' exercise on the Pincian mount, which is well sheltered from the cold winds, without being exposed to the direct influence of the sun's rays.

From what I have seen of the climate of this city, I am strongly inclined to think it a preferable situation, for the generality of consumptive patients, to those which are more generally recommended. The air has a softness that I never felt in the south of France, or at Nice ; and by those who believe such an atmosphere favourable in cases of pulmonary consumption, and prefer a situation removed some distance from the sea, Rome must have the preference.

The *Tramontana* is frequently felt at Rome with considerable severity, and during the winter, the climate is, without doubt, colder than that of Nice.

It is chiefly during the spring months, it appears to me, that Rome has the advantage in point of climate, being less liable to the keen cutting winds of the places I have already noticed. This is, however, an important circumstance, as the great difficulty is to find a good spring climate, for the consumptive patient ; the cold winds, which that season is liable to, I believe over the whole of Europe, being the evil most to be dreaded. At Naples they are particularly complained of. In truth, I believe no place is exempt from them ; nor must I be understood as stating Rome to be so : all I wish to be understood is, that Rome is less liable to these winds, than most places I have seen.

I met with a few cases at Rome rather favourable to the opinion I have ventured to give of it in consumptive cases. One gentleman, labouring under an affection of the lungs which rendered him very liable to attacks of inflammation in these organs, and who had several other symptoms, shewing, at least, a strong ten-

dency to Phthisis,' went to Naples during the
winter with the intention of stopping there some
time, but very soon after his arrival, he was
attacked with Hæmoptysis, and obliged to return to Rome, where he always feels comfortable.

Another gentleman, whose mother died of
an affection of the lungs, and who himself had
suffered long from Hæmoptysis followed by
cough, copious expectoration, &c., found much
benefit during a winter's residence at Rome,—his
cough, pain of chest, &c., having left him, and
he gained strength. In March he went to Naples,
when his symptoms soon began to return the
cough and pain of chest became troublesome, and
he felt a general irritability which prevented him
from sleeping.* He remained a month at Naples
and then returned to Rome, where these unpleasant symptoms very soon disappeared. This case
was related to me by the gentleman himself,
who, from having been long an invalid, had,
from necessity, paid particular attention to his
symptoms and the effects of climate upon them.

A lady who had lost several of her family
from consumption, who was subject to occasional
cough with an increased secretion from the
bronchiæ, at times tinged with blood, and was
a good deal emaciated, got rid of all her unpleasant symptoms during her residence at Rome,

* This gentleman always feels more or less of this when near the sea.

K

and even gained strength and flesh. This lady
had lost ground during the preceding winter
at Nice; and was one of those I alluded to, as
having been attacked with Hæmoptysis in the
spring.

These few cases appear to me worthy of remark; they afford but a slender evidence, it is
true, in favour of Rome, but they do afford some,
and of that kind, too, which we want most;
and I doubt much, whether the whole of the
climates recommended to, and frequented by,
our consumptive patients, in the south of France
and Italy, could bring forward as much in the
same space of time.

Should these observations ever be the means
of inducing a consumptive patient to go to
Rome, I must caution him to consider himself
strictly as an invalid, otherwise Rome is a dangerous residence.—He must not imagine that
he can enter with impunity into those amuse-
ments, from which he was prohibited at home.
The houses of Rome are not well calculated for
gaiety during winter; and, indeed, the same
remark is generally applicable to the houses all
over Italy. The stair-cases and lobbies are
large and open, and subject to currents of air,
of which invalids not unfrequently feel the
effects.

Many of the streets in Rome, too, are damp
and chilly, and the alternation between these
shaded streets, and situations exposed to the
sun is often very great. On this account the
open carriages, so much in use at Rome, are
very dangerous to the delicate, and close carriages should be alone used during the winter.
Neither must the invalid pass his time among
the ruins of the ancient city, nor the churches of
the modern,—both of which are frequently damp
and always cold,—until the season is so far
advanced as to make them safe for him. Ladies,
in particular, visiting these churches, should be
careful to protect themselves by warm thick
shoes from the extreme coldness of the marble
floors.

In these remarks on the churches I do not
include St. Peter's. From the immense body
of air which it contains, it is always of a mild
temperature, and always safe for the invalid.
On examining its temperature by the thermometer in January, I found it exactly 60°
(when the external air at 2 P. M. varied from
50°· to 55°·) which I imagine is very near the
medium annual temperature of Rome.* It is

* Since writing the above, I find by Professor Leslie's calculations
that the medium annual temperature of the latitude of Rome, calculated for the level of the sea, is exactly 60°. See Supplement to
Encyclopedia Britannica—Article ' Climate.'

commonly said that St. Peter's is hot in winter,
and cold in summer; the truth is the temperature of St. Peter's remains unchanged, and it
is the variations of the external air, and of our
sensations, at these seasons, that give rise to
the deception. During rainy weather when my
patients were deprived of exercise, 1 not unfrequently recommended a visit to this magnificent structure, where they found both occupation for the mind, and a mild temperature to
take exercise in.

By attention to these hints, 1 am inclined to
think the consumptive patient may pass the
winter at Rome fully as well as at any other part
of Italy, and perhaps better. The best residence is somewhere about the Piazza di Spagna,
which is well sheltered, and has the advantage
of being close to the Pincian Mount, which
affords the best protected and most delightful
walk at Rome. The Via Babuina is a bad
situation.

It is almost unnecessary to mention that accommodations are good and abundant in Rome.
The provisions in general are also very good;
and the fountains are not more famed for their
beauty, than estimable for the abundance and
purity of their water, which is brought from
a great distance.

Having finished the few observations I had to make on the climate of Rome, as far as it relates to the class of patients, which I have had chiefly in view,* a few remarks on the dreaded *Malaria* which of late years has excited so much attention, may not be thought misplaced here. They will be very general however, and are more intended for the popular than the medical reader. Neither my time nor opportunities admitted of that extensive enquiry and observation that could enable me to communicate much satisfactory information on this subject to the latter, though it is one which affords a very interesting field for investigation.

* There is one class of affections for which the Atmosphere of Rome appeared to me unfavourable—these are headaches arising from a tendency to fullness about the head. In many cases among the English residents, I found persons not previously subject to head aches affected with them here, and some already liable to them had them aggravated. Apoplexy, I was told, was at one time so frequent at Rome that a day of public fasting was ordered, and a particular form of prayer addressed to St. Anthony to avert so dreadful a calamity from the Holy City. This peculiarity of the climate of Rome has been also, I find, noticed by a native author.

Alexander de Petronius in his book De victu Romanorum, remarks (Lib. 4 cap. 1) " Itaque inter peculiares Urbis Romæ morbos, primus esse videtur multa succorum in capite exuberantia, quam destillationes plurimæ in subjectas partes sequuntur. Profecto hæc (si nomina fingere liceret) juxta id, quod caput plenum in hoc affectu sentitur, *capiplenium*, barbarè quidem, sed verè forsan, appellaremus. Hanc affectionem pauci qui Romam incolunt effugiunt."

Of the intimate nature of the causes of this fever we are entirely ignorant. That it generally proceeds from some noxious matter suspended in the air of the marshy grounds around Rome there appears little doubt. This is called ' *aria cattiva*', or bad air, by the inhabitants. It is not confined altogether to the low grounds, being found in some high situations; though in some of the instances of this I am inclined to believe that the aria cattiva is not generated on those spots, but gradually wafted thither by winds passing over the lower marshy lands.

And yet, when the circumstances that are favourable to its formation, or with which at least it seems generally to be present in the lower grounds, occur in the higher, such as stagnant water, marshy ground, or close damp situations,—all of which may be found in some parts of the Villa Borghese; in these cases we know no reason why it should not exist on the higher grounds as well as the lower; unless, indeed, it be, that the former are more exposed to winds which may be suposed to dilute and carry off the miasmata as quickly as formed : but even this is often prevented by the shelter of neighbouring trees.

Whatever be the source of this noxious quality in the air, it certainly seems to be gra-

dually extending itself in the neighbourhood of
Rome. Where it may end is difficult to say;
but, if we may credit an eloquent writer in the
Edinburgh Review,* and some late French
authors, such is the progress which it is making,
that the period seems not far distant when the
metropolis of the world will become a desert,
and the banks of the Tiber be shunned with as
much horror as they are now sought with eager-
ness by the enquiring and classic traveller. The
Romans themselves, however, smile at these
exaggerated reports.

Under such gloomy prospects for the inhabitants of this ill-fated country, it is some consolation to know that the numbers attacked by
this disease are not annually and progressively
increasing, as some writers would lead us to
believe, and as might be expected. This I was
assured of by several of the Roman Physicians,
and also by Signor Scaramucci, advocate and
secretary to the council for the general administration of hospitals.† This gentleman had paid
some attention to this subject, and, from making

* Edin. Rev. Vol. 28, p. 57.

† The direction of the Hospitals of Rome is intrusted to a general
administration as in Paris.

out the annual reports of these hospitals, could
speak correctly on it.

The *Malaria fever* occurs chiefly among the
inhabitants of the country at some distance from
Rome, who come down to the *Campagna* to
labour during the harvest; and the number of
fevers in the hospitals of Rome depends chiefly
on the state of the weather while these people
are employed in this task. If the season is dry
there are comparatively few fevers; if, on the
other hand, much rain falls, the hospitals are
much crowded. As these poor people are exposed to all the evils arising from hard labour
during such weather, and have the perspiration
frequently checked while flowing profusely, (a
sufficient cause alone, I believe, to produce
fever in many cases;) and as they pass the
night also on the very soil which gives birth to
the pernicious miasmata, it is not to be wondered that many should fall victims to such
concentrated causes. Among the inhabitants
of Rome who are more prudent, who never sleep
in the *Campagna*, but return to the city during
the night, the fever is comparatively rare. It is
in the summer and autumn that the *aria cattiva*
is most to be dreaded, and strangers arriving at
Rome in the autumn should not frequent the
places known to give rise to these fevers.—

Wherever there is stagnant water or marshy ground there is danger. Night is the most dangerous time to be exposed in these situations. The hours immediately after sun set, when the air is most loaded from the precipitation of the dew held in solution by the warmer air of the day, are also particularly dreaded by the Romans.

It has been supposed that the noxious effluvia are suspended in the atmosphere during the day in so diluted a state as generally to render them harmless, but being precipitated with the humidity of the air in the evening, they remain suspended in a more condensed state, and combined with the fresh vapours of the soil. Whether this explanation is just, or whether it is merely the greater degree of moisture in the atmosphere at this season of the day, which renders the noxious effluvia more active (as it certainly does render the impressions of odorous effluvia more sensible,) is of little consequence in our present enquiry : certain it is, however, that by far the greater proportion of those who are attacked by this fever, get it by exposure during the night.

It is also well known, that the best means of avoiding the danger, when obliged to pass

the night in infected places, are the use of fires
to keep the air dry, and getting as much above
the surface of the ground as possible,—a very
few feet having often been observed to mark the
line from safety to danger. A striking instance
of this was remarked to me by Professor BRERA,
(while going round the Clinical wards of the
Hospital of Padua with him) which is worth
recording as an additional proof to many that
are already in our possession.

The wall of that wing of the Hospital where
the clinical wards are, is washed by a branch
of the sluggish Brenta, and it has frequently hap-
pened that the windows of the men's ward
(which may be about sixteen feet above the surface of the water) having been carelessly left
open till too late an hour, several of the patients
have been attacked with intermittent fevers, in
some instances of the pernicious kind.[*]

This has never occurred in the women's
wards, which are immediately over those of the
men, though there is no reason to believe that
more care was taken in shutting the windows of
them than of the men's wards

---

[*] If the observations of Dr. Regaud are correct, gauze frames
fitted to these windows, while they admitted the air would arrest the
progress of the Miasmata ; this precaution might be useful in all cases
where windows are exposed directly to the air of marshes.

When at Florence in June last, I met with two young gentlemen, who, in passing the Pontine marshes, had stopped during the night at an inn where the accommodations were not particularly inviting. One slept on the floor of a barn among some hay, with the door open. On his arrival at Florence, soon after, this gentleman was attacked by violent fever, which Dr. Downe, who has had extensive experience in the fevers of this climate, treated by copious depletion. Under this judicious treatment it soon put on the regular tertian type and yielded readily to bark. His companion, who had slept in the carriage, probably owed his safety in a great measure to his greater height above the surface of the ground placing him beyond the influence of the *aria cattiva*, which at this season (April) is not very active.*

The fevers of the winter and spring are generally only relapses of those of the preceding

---

* I have sometimes thought that the lives of many of the mountaineers, that come to work during harvest in the Campagna, might be saved by the erection for them of wooden houses elevated fifteen or twenty feet above the surface by means of wooden posts,—as they *will* sleep there notwithstanding the known danger. This might easily be done in a country where wood is plentiful ; and the advantages likely to be derived from it would be increased by the constant use of fires to windward through the night.

autumn. There appears no ground to apprehend
an attack of Malaria fever at Rome, from the
first of November till June, and not even afterwards if the dangerous places are avoided. This
fever in its nature differs but little from fevers
arising under similar circumstances in all warm
countries.   The Jungle fever of India,—the
fevers of the coast of Africa,—of the Spanish
Main ; the Malaria fever of Italy,—the Yellow
fever of the West Indies, &c.,* are probably all
children of the same family, originating from
similar causes, and modified only by the peculiar circumstances under which they show themselves. The Malaria fevers are mostly of the
tertian type, appearing in all the different degrees of severity from the mild regular tertian,
to what are called pernicious, generally accompanied with a degree of coma, which not unfrequently would prove fatal in a few paroxysms
but for the speedy administration of large doses
of bark.

* And according to some late observations perhaps the plague
itself. London Medical Repository, December 1817.

During the summers of 1818 and 1819, the *malaria* fevers were more generally and severely felt than usual ; and this has been entirely owing to the very unseasonable fall of rain in both these years. In ordinary years, the intermittent .fevers of Rome are, as I have said, produced by the marshy grounds in its vicinity, and the inhabitants never fail to be affected by them in a greater or less degree ; but when rains fall early in the summer, the sources of the noxious miasmata are greatly extended, and come home, in some places, to the very thresholds of the Romans,—occasioning, necessarily, a proportionate increase of the numbers attacked by the disease.

These additional sources of danger are to be found in the stagnant waters, saturated with vegetable substances, formed intentionally, or allowed to accumulate, in the gardens of Rome ; and in the masses of vegetable matters left to putrefy at every corner, even in the very streets, —all of which only require a sufficient supply of heat and moisture to prove abundantly pernicious. From this—certainly remediable—evil, some of the ' *saluberrimi colles*' have lost all claim to that epithet during the malaria season. But this is nothing new : the same thing occurred formerly.—TheEsquiline itself, when Rome was

*M

nearly in its most populous condition, and when
this hill was in a neglected state, and used only
as a Cemetery for the common people, (until
Mæcenas cleared it of its rubbish and formed
his gardens there) proved a plentiful source of
disease.*

The same causes that are now so productive
of these periodical fevers at Rome, probably
always existed, in a greater, or less degree,
and were always followed by similar effects.
This is very evident from the excuses offered
by Horace in one of his epistles to Mæcenas
(Epist. vii. Lib. i.) for not having returned to
the city according to his promise. He writes
in the end of August, or beginning of September,
and characterises, in the following very striking
terms, the unhealthy nature of the preceding
period :—

———— dum ficus prima, calorque
Designatorem decorat lictoribus atris ;
Dum pueris omnis pater et matercula pallet ;
Officiosaque sedulitas, et opella forensis
Adducit febres, et testamenta resignat.

* " L' Esquilino insino a tanto che servì di cimeterio alla
plebe Romana abdondó di mefitiche esalazioni, e poco fu abitato :
ma a tempo d'Augosto ne fu megliorata l'aria per opera principalmente
di Mecenate, chi vi stabilì i suoi orti con una magnifica abitazione, per
cui vi concorse ad abitare molta altra gente." Dissertazione sul culto
reso dagli antichi Romani alla Dea Febre—Del Dottor G. De
Matthæis p. 35. This original insalubrity, and its removal by Mæcenas, are noticed by Horace in Sat. vii Lib. 1.

" Nunc licet Esquiliis habitare salubribus, &c."

Those destructive fevers, also, that Livy and some other Authors speak of, which at different times raged at Rome, were, in all probability, no other than the *malaria* fevers of the present day ; at least, after much research on this subject, this is the opinion of my learned friend professor De Matthæis, who, in the classical dissertation already referred to, observes at page 27— " Le tante pestilenze, che, al referire di Tito Livio, hanno cosi spesso assalita e desolata questa citta, non possono essere state che epidemie di febbri di tal natura *(periodical fevers,)* la di cui causa ordinaria debb' essere stata accresciuta e renforzata dalle particolari costituzioni annuali."

Were there a medical police established at Rome, (and no city has more need of one) much might be done for the mitigation of this evil. Were all stagnant waters removed from their gardens, were these and the vineyards, &c. carefully drained to prevent the formation of more,—were all decaying vegetable and animal substances removed, and were their streets kept clean and dry,— there would be fewer *malaria* quarters in Rome. If they are unable to drain the marshes, by a little exertion they might, at least, keep their invisible enemy without the gates.

Yet even in the most unhealthy seasons the fever period only continues during the summer

months, and the fears of strangers visiting Rome,
on account of *malaria*, after October, are, as I have
already observed, without grounds. Among the
numbers of English in Italy last year I did not
hear of, nor do I believe that there was, one attacked with this fever from October to June,—the
solitary instance excepted, which I have noticed
in a former page as having occurred in April. In
this case, the individual, it will be seen, exposed
himself in the most imprudent manner.

From the exaggerated reports that had gone
abroad of the uncommon prevalence of fever at
Rome during the summer of 1819, and from the
circumstance of an English physician having died
of it,* many English travellers were deterred from
coming on to Rome in the end of autumn. On
my arrival however, at Rome, early in November, I found the hospitals nearly cleared of these
fevers, and it will be seen directly that the actual
number of attacks during this season was considerably less than in the preceding year.

The following is an abstract of the whole
number of *malaria* fevers, (with their result) received into the great hospital of Santo Spirito
during the two last seasons. This hospital is,

---

* My excellent friend Dr. Slaney.

beyond all comparison, the largest in Rome; it is wholly appropriated to male patients, the far greater proportion of whom are Peasants, who get the fever while labouring in the Campagna, as I have already remarked.

	Received.	Died
1818	8137	363
1819	6134	258

This statement shows the numbers attacked to be, certainly, very great, and also the proportion of deaths; though both are much less than the exaggerated reports of some of our travellers would lead us to believe. It is to be recollected, too, that these are the numbers in two very sickly seasons, and that, during the months of their prevalence, these fevers form almost the sole diseases that are met with in Rome:—August is the month in which the greatest number of patients are received. The proportional mortality has been somewhat greater this season, 1819, than last, and the sequelæ, which are chiefly obstructions of the abdominal viscera, more frequent than usual.

Bark is the sole remedy employed in Rome for these fevers, and the quantity taken by some individuals during the season is immense. The Prince of Peace, who resided at Rome last

year, took six pounds, and I am acquainted
with an English gentleman, who has been long
resident in Rome, and who has suffered severely
from the fever this year, having had repeated
relapses, who, during the present season has
taken thirteen pounds, the whole in substance!
I was curious to know the quantity consumed
at the Santo Spirito during the last two seasons,
and found, on enquiry, that it amounted in 1818,
to 3200 pounds, and in 1819, to 2960 pounds!

There is a strong prejudice against the employment of the arseniate of Potass or Soda,
though I have no doubt, that, in many of the
more tedious cases, one or other of these preparations might be employed with much advantage, and perfect safety. I suggested the trial
of one of them to an English physician here,
who had long suffered under tertian notwithstanding the diligent use of the bark :—he took
the pure oxide in an extremely small quantity,
sufficient, however, to excite slight nausea, and
it at once stopped the fever. Some of the Alkaline Salts, particularly the Carbonate of
Potass, and Muriate of Ammonia are joined
frequently, in small quantities, to the bark, but
the preparations of mercury are scarcely ever
used. In the cases that I have met with among
the Romans, which were chiefly cases of relapse

in servants in English families, I think I have
observed benefit from the use of calomel purgatives previous to administering the bark. I
was naturally led to the employment of these
from the sallow countenances, and yellow eyes
of the patients, and from their known utility, in
such cases, in English practice; and in one
case, to the surprise of an Italian Lady, a
couple of purgatives cured her of her fever.

The cases of intermittent that occur during
winter and spring, are, as I have before remarked, almost entirely relapses, and it frequently occurs that in the acute diseases of these
seasons, in subjects who during the preceding
autumn have had intermittent, that the fever attending their present disease—let it be rheumatism, pleurisy, or any other inflammatory affection,—assumes the intermittent form, requiring,
when the inflammatory symptoms are removed,
the employment of the bark. A case of this
kind was pointed out to me in the hospital of
St. John. The combination here was with
acute rheumatism, affecting chiefly one knee,
and the case proved speedily fatal by the super-
vention of gangrene of the limb.

Cernis ut e molli sanguis pulmone refluxus
Ad Stygias certo limine ducat aquas.

In every climate, and under all circumstances, pulmonary consumption, when once
fully formed, I fear will be found to justify the
character given of it by Ovid, who, doubtless,
had this disease in view, when he wrote the
above lines. Its course may be more or less
rapid, but its termination is ever the same.
At Rome, this disease is not unfrequent, yet
it is far from being one of their most prominent
maladies, as at Marseilles and Genoa. Neither
is it so rapid in its progress in general, as in
these places, though, in this respect, there is
much variety : two years, from the most accurate
information I could obtain, appear to be about
its average duration.

The treatment of consumption at Rome,
and some other parts of Italy, as far as regards
the supposed utility of a sea or land atmosphere, shews, in a very striking point of view,
the discrepancy in the opinions of medical men
on this subject. The physicians on the sea-coast,
send their patients into the interior of the
country, and those in the interior to the shores
of the Mediterranean or Adriatic, according
as they fancy the air of the one or the other

preferable. From Genoa they send their consumptive patients into the interior, deeming the
sea-air injurious to them. From Naples they
frequently send such patients, and for similar
reasons, to Rome. From Rome, on the other
hand, they send their consumptive cases frequently to Cività Vécchia, on the shores of the
Mediterranean ; more frequently to the shores of
the Adriatic, and occasionally even to Naples.
Formerly Galen and Celsus sent such patients
to Egypt; but, probably, in this case, the voyage
was considered as of more importance than the
change of air.

This variety of practice either shews that
neither a sea nor land air is best fitted to all
cases of consumption, or rather, I fear, that
both are equally ineffectual. These migrations
are continued chiefly from habit, for none of
the medical men seemed to expect much benefit
from them ; indeed most of those with whom
I had communication on the subject seemed
unable to give an opinion whether the change,
whatever it might be, was of any use or not.
All appear to agree in the preference to be given
to a mild and equable climate (which is no where
to be found), and all whose opinions I have
heard, prefer a low situation, and rather a
humid than dry atmosphere.

*N

In the hospitals of Rome, particular wards
are set apart for consumptive patients,—a very
cruel practice, and originating in the old, and
almost obsolete opinion of the contagious nature of this disease; an opinion, like almost
all other popular ones relating to diseases,
originating with medical men themselves, and
maintained by the vulgar (long after they have
been laid aside, from a conviction of their error,
by the former) and too often, as in the present instance, to the injury of the unfortunate patient.—
The consumptive ward of the Santo Spirito,
which contained eleven beds, had, at my visit,
only three patients. I observed several of the
bed-steads covered with piles of bed-clothes,
which, I was informed, had been sent there by
the friends of consumptive patients who had
died, from an idea that it was dangerous to
use them afterwards *

As corroborative of the opinion I have given
of the disease of the lungs described by Dr.

* The very generally prevalent opinion of the common people on
the continent of the contagious nature of consumption I have already
noticed, but I was not a little surprized to hear lately that the clinical
professor of one of the French Universities strongly maintains the same
opinion, and still more so to hear some of the instances he gave in support of it.

Sinclair as occurring in the Mediterranean fleet, I may add that of Dr. de Matthæis, Professor of Medicine in the Sapienza of Rome, which is exactly that which I stated before, viz: that the disease described by this gentleman is very different from the disease properly designated under the name of pulmonary consumption, both in England and Italy. The latter is a disease originating most commonly, as is well known, in causes inherent in the constitution of the individuals attacked, comparatively slow in its progress, and exhibiting not only, certainly in England and Italy, but I believe, also, in all other climates, symptoms very different from those described by Dr. Sinclair.

In the disease described by him, the lungs are attacked without any previous constitutional tendency to consumption, by acute and violent inflammation, which, if not speedily arrested in its progress, terminates in the disorganization of these organs, and the consequent death of the patient. Inflammations of the lungs, having a similar termination, are by no means unfrequent on the Italian shores of the Mediterranean, though certainly less so than they are described to have been in our Mediterranean fleet, and this is perhaps a sufficient proof that some of the causes of the frequency of the disease

among our sailors, must have depended on
some particular circumstances in the life of the
individual, and cannot be wholly attributable
to the climate. It is but justice to Dr. Sinclair
to observe, that Professor de Matthæis (who
read Dr. S.'s Thesis) gives him every credit for
describing with accuracy the progress of inflammation of the lungs, such as he acknowledges
to be of frequent occurrence in the Italian
peninsula.

NAPLES.

Though the plan I laid down for myself was to give some account of the places only which I visited; it may be expected that, in a work of this kind, some notice should be taken of a place like Naples, which has been so often recommended, and so often tried, in pulmonary consumption. Of it I can only speak from the report of others, but from a good deal of attention to the subject, and from conversations with medical men who had visited it, I think I shall not be far wrong in stating the climate of Naples to come very near that of Nice, nearer at least, than to any other climate we have mentioned.

It has the same cloudless skies, the same powerful sun, and comparative great warmth during the winter months, and is subject to similar cutting winds during the spring. So much indeed are the latter felt, that I have heard it as a remark by some of the Italians themselves, that Naples was the warmest situation in Italy during the winter, and coldest during the spring. Though this is not to be taken in the literal sense, it shows forcibly the

striking difference of these two seasons. The
same similarity which exists between the climates of Naples and Nice, I am afraid also exists
between their effects on pulmonary consumption.
I have never yet met one medical man, or consumptive invalid, who had been there, who gave
a good report of it, while I have met several
who gave a bad one. Among others my friend
Dr. Heath, who passed the winter of 1818 and
1819 at Naples, informed me that the climate
certainly did not appear to him to agree with
the consumptive patients that came under his
observation while there.

ON A SUMMER RESIDENCE.

I have now finished the observations I had to offer on the subject of a winter's residence for patients labouring under pulmonary consumption ; and it only remains to make a few remarks on the situations best suited as a summer residence, for those who remain more than one winter abroad, This is not a matter of indifference. It is a question often asked by such patients, and proves one of more difficult solution than might at first sight appear. ,

It is more easy to say what such a residence should not be, than what it should. The situations recommended as most favourable for winter residences are improper during the summer ; the very circumstances to which they owe their mildness during the former season, rendering them oppressively hot in the latter. I believe I shall not err, if I say that the whole of the south of France and Italy are improper for consumptive patients during the summer months,*

---

* That there may not be some cool spots in both these countries, (and I shall immediately mention one) where such patients might pass the summer as well as elsewhere I am not prepared to say ; my remarks refer only to those places known and resorted to by strangers.

and that the more certainly, the farther the
disease is advanced: where hectic fever is formed, and ulceration of the lungs has taken place,
a high temperature certainly accelerates the
progress of the disease.

Dr. Sinclair, in the work formerly quoted,
states that August and September in the Mediterranean are very fatal to patients labouring
under pulmonary consumption ; and that those
taken ill in March and April rarely outlive the
great heats and noxious winds of the succeeding
summer.* The months of January and February,
when the temperature is steady, are stated by
this gentleman to be the only months when consumptive patients can remain with safety in the
Mediterranean or on its shores.

Though I do not think the observations of
Dr. Sinclair are quite conclusive against the
good effects of the climate of the Mediterranean
and its shores on the generality of cases of pulmonary consumption which occur in England,
and are sent abroad to pass the winter months
only, they certainly show the impropriety of
such patients remaining in that climate during
the heats of summer,—an observation which I

---

* Dr. S. alludes particularly to the sirocco, during the prevalence
of which he observed consumptive complaints much aggravated.

have found corroborated by all the medical men of my acquaintance who have had opportunity of judging.

It is rather a singular circumstance that while the English practitioners were sending their consumptive patients to the shores of the Mediterranean, our naval medical officers navigating that sea were sending theirs to England. Whether an attention to the difference of season which such advice had, or ought to have had in view, would not, in some measure, reconcile the apparent contradiction, I shall leave others to judge.

The same injurious effects in hurrying on the fatal termination of consumption, after ulceration had commenced, have been communicated to me by many of my naval friends who had served in the West Indies, as uniformly observed there. And I know that a practice formerly prevalent in the navy of sending seamen affected with this disease to that country, in the hope of obtaining an alleviation of their complaints, has been of late years abandoned, owing to the representation of the naval medical officers of that country. From these facts, and also from my own observations in the countries themselves, I can have no doubt, nor indeed, do I believe, is there any doubt, of the impropriety of con-

M

sumptive patients remaining in the south of France and Italy during the heats of summer. This is a circumstance, however, which has not been sufficiently attended to by medical men in directing such patients in the choice of a residence.

When I was at Florence in the end of May last, I met with a young gentleman labouring under pulmonary consumption, who had just been sent from England to Italy by his physician. At this time the heat was beginning to get oppressive, and this poor young man already began to feel the effect of it in the increased profusion of his night sweats. Dr. Downe, who was well aware of the effects of the summer in Italy in such cases, very properly advised him to retrace his steps, and get beyond the Alps as speedily as he could. This case also affords another example of the vague, and too often erroneous advice given to such patients on leaving their own country.

The only part of Italy which I have seen, where it appears to me that such patients as could not conveniently leave it, might pass the summer, is on the banks of the Lake of Como. About Cadenabbia, or rather on the opposite shore, twenty-five miles up the Lake, I should think the best situation. Here, sheltered by the hills from the intense heat of the summer's

sun, and enjoying all the advantages which this
beautiful lake affords him, the invalid, strolling
along its banks, or gliding over the surface of its
lucid waters, with the view of either exercise or
amusement, might, I think, pass a few months
safely and pleasantly.*

The most common practice, however, and
perhaps the best, is for those who have passed
the winter in Italy, and mean to return thither,
to go to Switzerland during the summer. This
country is assuredly by no means free from faults
as a residence for consumptive patients. On the
contrary, its climate is very variable, and requires
much care on the part of the patient and his
attendants; yet, all things considered, it is probably the best one accessible to the invalid.
The part of Switzerland most frequented by
the English is the vicinity of the Lake of Geneva;
and, probably, as good a situation may be
found in this neighbourhood as in any part of
the country. Vevey, situated at the eastern
extremity of the lake, though the mildest
climate perhaps in the whole of Switzerland

* Pliny's Fountain, on the banks of this Lake, which was flowing
very copiously when I examined it (June 20th), sunk the thermometer
to 50°, while the temperature of the Lake was 60°, and of the air in
the shade at noon 70°. For an account of this singular fountain see
Eustace's Classical Tour.

during winter, is not the most favourable for a
summer residence. Those probably best calculated as such, and certainly those most commonly selected, are Lausanne and Geneva, of
which I shall now give some account.

Lausanne lies high and rather exposed to the
bize, a cold dry north-east wind, which is frequently felt with a good deal of severity, especially in the evenings, in this country. The
bize often alternates with a southerly wind during the day. In choosing a residence in this
neighbourhood particular regard should be had
to this circumstance. The climate of Geneva
is cold during the winter, its situation greatly
exposing it to the same cold winds. In the
neighbourhood of both these places, however,
particular spots may be selected, which will
answer very well for summer residences. In the
neighbourhood of Geneva the most favourable
is on the northern side of the Lake ; but the
town itself ought not to be chosen as a residence.
Near Lausanne the most favourable situations
are to be found on the low grounds near the
margin of the lake. Here, indeed, the heat
during the forenoon is frequently inconvenient ;
yet, upon the whole, it affords the best residence, being that which is the most effectually
sheltered from the bize.

With a little attention, then, to the choice of a sheltered situation, I have no doubt that the consumptive invalid may pass the summer on the banks of this lake as well as in any part of Switzerland. In addition to the agreeable abode and beautiful country in which he resides, he is well situated for returning to Italy at the proper season. The journey to Switzerland, is no doubt rather a long one ; but if care is taken to leave Italy before the summer heat becomes oppressive, and to return before the cold weather sets in in Switzerland, it may be comfortably performed, as far as climate is concerned, and in some cases, perhaps, with advantage to the patient from the journey.* The invalid may arrive in Switzerland by the middle of June, and leave it towards the latter end of September.

* In travelling, the torpid state into which all the chylopoetic viscera generally fall, often produces much inconvenience to patients with any febrile symptoms, and such patients should be provided against it. This very general effect of travelling led me to expect benefit from it in a case of diarrhœa, accompanying hectic fever in a consumptive patient, and, on account of it, I willingly allowed the patient to make a journey of several days. The effect was much more than I anticipated : a diarrhœa which for six weeks all the usual medicines had failed in checking for more than one day at a time, yielded completely to this short journey, without any other evident cause, and even a degree of constipation supervened. The Diarrhœa did not return for several months. There are some kinds of this disease where the effect of carriage exercise continued for several days, might preve of much benefit .

The passage of the Alps, which may be either made by the Simplon or Mont Cenis, the roads over both being good, often dwells upon the mind of the invalid, and not unfrequently on that of his medical attendant, as fraught with no little danger. But I have already said, that, if passed at the proper season, there is no ground for this apprehension. They may be crossed with perfect safety at any time from June to October; and this is perhaps restricting the time to shorter limits than necessary. The invalid leaving Switzerland for Italy would do well to commence his journey towards the end of September. I have twice crossed the Simplon in the end of June, and found the weather extremely pleasant, only rather warm during the forenoon. I also crossed this mountain once on the 9th and 10th of October. In ascending it at this time it was very warm, and even at the highest point (though a little snow had fallen a few days before,) not by any means very cold. At the village of Simplon, a little beyond the summit, and probably five or six hundred feet lower, on the evening of the 9th after sun-set, the thermometer stood at 42°, and, at sun-rise the following morning, at 41°. The inn of the Simplon is good, and an invalid will find himself more

comfortably lodged and better entertained than
in a large proportion of the inns on the road.
I am the more particular in stating this, because
I have heard doubts expressed by medical men
about the propriety of allowing a consumptive
patient to pass the night in such a mountain.
Nothing, in my opinion, can be more absurd.
The invalid who is capable of passing the Simplon at all, may sleep here with perfect safety,
and get over his journey much more comfortably
than by crossing the mountain in one day, by
doing which he will require to sit about eleven
successive hours in his carriage.

As in the account of other places, of which I
have already spoken, I shall now say something
of the diseases and medical practice in this
country.

At Lausanne there is a small general hospital
in the town, forming part of the workhouse, and
also a small lunatic asylum a little out of town,
where every comfort that the nature of the building admits is paid to the patients.

The only thing I observed worthy of remark
in the general hospital was a plan of treating
fractures by suspending the fractured limb, as
first recommended and described by Dr. Sauter
of Constance. Mr. Major the very intelligent

surgeon of this hospital, has translated Dr.
Sauter's work into French, and he uses the plan
with the greatest success. I feel quite convinced, from the cases that I saw under this
gentleman's charge, and from a careful examination of his very simple apparatus, that the
practice only requires to be fully known to come
into general use, in a great proportion of fractures,—particularly in compound ones,—with an
increase of comfort to the patient, and a diminution of attendance on the part of the surgeon.
The great advantage of suspending the limb in
this manner is, that it follows all the motions
of the body without the least danger of de-
ranging the fractured parts. A patient with a
fractured leg treated on this plan may get out of
bed and seat himself on a neighbouring one till
his own is prepared.* There are several other
affections of the extremities in which this plan
of suspension might be adopted, such as violent
inflammations, gout, &c.†

* In my late visit to England I was informed that some account of
this work is given in the medical and physical journal.

† Vide Nuovo e piu semplice Metodo di curare le Fratture degli
arti. Milan 1817.

Pulmonary consumption is a frequent disease
in this country. In a conversation that I had
with professor Jurine of Geneva, a gentleman of
extensive experience in affections of the chest, I
found he preferred keeping his patients in their
rooms at a regulated temperature, to sending
them to Nice, which latter practice he thinks
rather an injurious one. He uses the inhalations
of the steam of warm water in some affections
of the lungs with much benefit, particularly in
cases of long continued expectoration, accompanied with irritability and sleeplessness; and
he stated to me several cases of this kind, in
support of his observation. He is of opinion
that remedies used in the way of inhalation are
too little attended to. He uses an inhaler with
a very large neck, and an opening at the end
sufficiently large to admit the patient's mouth,
so that he may inhale the steam without any
exertion. In one case he has found inhaling the
vapour of pitch and rosin very useful in abating
the expectoration; the patient uses it an hour
or two every day, and has done so for many
years.

Sporadic cases of fever are not uncommon
at Geneva, but contagious fevers are rare. In
the convalescence from Scarlatina the medi-

cal men of this place are particularly careful in guarding their patients from exposure to cold; the general rule being not to suffer such patients to leave their rooms for six weeks. Dropsical affections are what they seem to dread most. On what the greater danger in such cases depends here I could not learn; but from what I heard and observed in several instances, it appeared to me that the seqaelæ of this disease are more severely felt in Switzerland than with us.

A medicine in very general use in Geneva, and which I believe is scarcely known among us, is the sugar of milk, 'Saccho-Lactic acid'. It is prepared in large quantities in some parts of the country, and is brought to the apothecary in crystallized cakes; all he does is to reduce it to a powder. It is given in the dose of from two or three drams to an ounce or more. Its taste is by no means disagreeable, its operation is said to be very mild, and it remains on the stomach often when other medicines are rejected. The mode of preparation of this salt is very simple, consisting merely in the evaporation of whey to the point of crystallization, dissolving the salt afresh, for the purpose of purification, and then finally crystallizing a second time.

If this medicine supports the character given
me of it, I should think it might be introduced
with advantage into the list of our saline purgatives, and would probably supersede some of
them, from its being free from the disagreeable
nauseous taste of the latter, and sitting so easily
on the stomach. The trials I have myself made
of it are not sufficient to warrant my giving any
very decided opinion of its effects.

Much good fellowship and reciprocal communication exist among the medical men of
Geneva. They are also extremely liberal in
their intercourse with strangers, who seldom
fail to leave their society without increasing
their knowledge and receiving many marks of
attention. They have several societies or meetings. The physicians and surgeons have each
their own once a week ; and once a fortnight
there is a general meeting of members in all
classes of the profession. The fatal cases, and
any interesting cases that have occurred in the
intervals of the meetings are related.*

From meetings conducted as these appeared
to me to be, much advantage cannot fail to be

---

* No body is interred at Geneva till it is examined by a medical
man particularly appointed by the government.

derived by the medical men themselves, and the
community of which they are members.   At one
of these meetings at which I had the pleasure
to be present, Dr. Pecher related a case which
had occurred in his practice a few days before,
of a woman who had lately fallen into a low
melancholy state without any evident cause;
the day after he saw her she complained of uneasiness about the stomach, and on the next
fell into syncope, which continued a considerable time   Soon after this she passed per anum
upwards of two handfuls of hard concretions,
which from the appearance of one presented to
the society appeared to me to be biliary calculi.*

I may here notice a singular practice followed in this country in consumption and some
other affections, of eating large quantities of
ripe grapes during the autumn. About Lausanne
and Vevey the finest grapes of Switzerland are
produced, and the inhabitants from other parts
of the country often go there to pass a few weeks
among the vineyards. They purchase a portion

---

* One of these was given to Berzelius the celebrated Swedish
Chemist, then at Geneva, to analize ; and I mentioned the circumstance
the following day to Dr. Marcet, who will no doubt attend to it, as
connected with his philosophical and excellent work on calculou
disorders.

of one that they may have the grapes when they choose, and each individual generally eats several pounds a day. The reports I had of this practice were not of that correct kind to enable me to draw any satisfactory conclusion on its effects. That such a practice should be continued and repeated annually, by many persons, without some advantage being derived from it, is at least unlikely ; but I fear much is not to be expected from it in consumption. And yet from their cooling subacid nature, ripe grapes may deserve a trial, where the patient has an opportunity. To expect much use from them, however, they ought, I apprehend, to form a large proportion of the diet of the patient. In this way, continued for a considerable time, they may favour the removal of obstructions. Dr. Moore relates two cases of evident pulmonary consumption, of which the subjects, by living several months in Switzerland on ripe grapes and bread, seemed to derive much advantage.*

Before leaving the subject of Switzerland, I must not forget to caution those who are subject to inflammatory affections of the chest, not to attempt ascending the mountains of that coun-

* Travels in France and Italy.

try. By this practice they are often thrown into a violent perspiration, through the exertion necessary for the ascent and the exposure to a warm sun ; and the moment they reach the summit they are subjected to the influence of a cold air, which, together with the cessation from exercise, is fraught with much danger to such subjects.

CRETINISM. I may in this place, as well as in any other, introduce some observations I have to make on the subject of Cretinism.

On my way from Italy to Switzerland I had an opportunity of examining these wretched creatures, who are numerous in some parts of the Vallais, particularly in the centre, and about Sion the capital. In a small village in this neighbourhood, remarkable for the occurrence of cretins, and which is built in a low close and damp situation, I found, among many other instances, the whole of one family, amounting to four, in this shocking state of ideotism. The parents were healthy-looking people, and apparently free from any complaint. In some cases I found these poor creatures afflicted with cutaneous diseases, and others had nearly lost their sight from chronic inflammation.

Nothing can be more unsightly than the whole aspect of the Cretin. His diminutive stature, (which rarely exceeds four feet, and is often less at maturity,) his sluggish feeble motions, the large pendulous goitre which often accompanies this state, the sallow sickly complexion, coarse skin, deformed countenance approaching to that of the lower animals, his large mouth, thick coarse lips and eye lids, with the vacant and unmeaning stare and hideous grin which are often superadded on the approach of a stranger,—altogether compose a very shocking picture of humanity.

Cretinism exists in all the different degrees from the greatest stupidity up to perfect ideotism. Indeed the greater part of the inhabitants of the Vallais appeared to me to have an extremely heavy stupid appearance; and from all the information I could obtain, this seems truly to be no incorrect indication of the state of their mental faculties. I was pleased to find that this shocking disease is evidently decreasing in the valley, as well as goitres; particularly among the higher classes, who could send their children up to the mountains : and indeed it appears to me not unlikely that if the villages situated in the low close marshy situations, where this disease is most frequently met with, were destroyed, and the inhabitants removed to elevated dry situations, the human form

would soon cease to be exhibited under so de-
graded an aspect.*

The causes of Cretinism and of Goitre—
Bronchocele—(which, though frequently accompanying the former, is not, as some defini-
tions of cretinism state, essential to its existence,) are far from being thoroughly accounted
for. Professor Foderé, who has written by far
the most learned work on Goitre and Cretinism,
brings forward numerous observations to shew
that both are produced by living in a humid
warm atmosphere in mountainous countries,
and that the idea of snow-water, hard water,
bad food, &c. being causes is entirely without
foundation. Dr. Foderé's opinion is founded on
very careful and extensive observations among
the vallies of the Alps, in one of which he was
born, and the opportunities I have had of examining these vallies lead me to agree in most
respects with him, and this indeed before I ever
saw his work. That the causes of goitre and
cretinism are the same, there can be little doubt.
Dr. F. says that goitrous parents, living in a

---

* A few excellent remarks on Cretinism will be found in Dr. Duncan's medical and surgical journal, Vol. V. by the late Dr. Reeve of
Norwich.

country where goitre is endemic, after two gene-
rations, not only have goitrous chidren, but
even cretins. Cretins are never found but where
goitres exist, though the latter are often found
without goitres ; yet this seems only to show
that a more powerful application of the common
cause is necessary to produce cretinism. In
the upper part of the Vallais, which is more
elevated, dry and open, goitres are rare, but in
the lower, more confined, and humid situations,
half the population appear goitrous, and cretins
are numerous : again, on first entering the mountains of Savoy, a few goitres may be remarked ;
on continuing the journey, and getting among
the Alps, at Aguibelle for example, at the entrance
of the valley of La Maurienne, surrounded with
mountains, goitres are common, a fifth of the
inhabitants perhaps being affected by them ; yet
I was told no cretins existed. In this place,
however, I saw several wandering about in a state
of demi-cretinism ; the diminutive size—the slow
feeble slouching gait—the half-formed cretin features—and the heedless stupid stare—all shewing that they were but one step removed from
perfect imbecility. Proceeding farther along this
valley, we come to St. Jean still more completely
embosomed in the high Alps, and here we find
a diminutive sallow population, goitres very fre-

quent, and often of a large size, and cretins common.   Thus as the supposed cause becomes more
powerful, goitres from being rare become frequent, and an approach to cretinism appears.

In France, among the Cevennes, the Vosges,
and the Soissonnais mountains, goitres are very
common, but cretins very rare.   On entering the
valley of Maurienne a close approach to cretinism
is added to goitre, and deeper in the same valley
both goitre and cretinism appear in the highest
degree.   Proceeding still farther up this valley
till we come to Lanslebourg, at the foot of
Mount Cenis, which though still surrounded by
higher mountains, is much more elevated (about
400 toises) than St. Jean, we find, as in the higher
part of the Vallais, both goitres and cretins dis-
appear ; for on enquiry at this place, I was told
there were neither, and on examination, I could
see neither.

Most infants that are to become cretins are
born with a small goitre.   Such infants are little
sensible, heavy, sleep much, and are easily distinguished from other children.   They are mostly
deaf and dumb, yet (apparently in attempting to
speak) they make a very disagreeable noise.   Dr.
Foderé observes, that cretins are generally long

lived, and little subject to disease, being entirely
exempt from the numerous class of maladies, to
which their fellow beings of a superior order are
subjected, those, namely, arising from affections
of the mind, and irregularities of living.

After all, I believe, it is much easier to trace
the *habitat* of these diseases, than to ascertain
their actual causes. Foderé, Saussure, and others,
certainly bring forward many strong arguments
in favour of the opinion that they derive their
origin from the moist, hot, and stagnating atmosphere of Alpine Vallies ; but, on the other hand,
Ramond, in his observations on the Pyrenées,
informs us that cretinism and goitre exist among
these mountains, even in greater extent and degree
than in the Vallais, and under circumstances of
locality very different, namely, in open, well-
watered, and well-ventilated vallies.

The common notion of snow-water being the
cause of this disease, is set at rest for ever by the
fact of its existing in countries (for instance Sumatra,) where snow is never found. Stronger arguments in favour of the opinion that traces it to
mineral or other impregnations of water, exist ;
and of these, the strongest I have met with is re-
corded in the Dict. des Sciences Medicales, article
Eau ; but this idea is certainly contradicted, and
confuted by numerous well established facts.

On my way south, I first observed the goitres
very frequent in Lyons.   In Provence I also met
with a few.   On approaching the Alps on the
Italian side they began to appear.   In the Vallais
they were particularly common,   through the
whole of Switzerland I found them frequent, and
I did not lose sight of them till after crossing
Les Vosges mountains, which divide Alsace from
the rest of France*

This   complaint   is   much   more   common
among women than men.   The tumour has been
observed also to augment during pregnancy, and
suppression of the senses has appeared as an ex-

---

* Cretinism is by no means confined to Europe, and still less
goitre : Thus Staunton, Marsden, Turner, Park, and more lately
Bowditch, &c. give an account of the great prevalence of this unsightly
degeneration in Chinese Tartary, Thibet, Sumatra, the interior of
Africa, and other countries approaching more or less in their local con-
figuration to its great European habitats.   The well known expression
of the Roman Satyrist—" Quis tumidum guttur miratur in Alpibus ?"
still retains its topographical propriety, and probably points out the
origin of the common name of the disease,—*goitre* being considered
by many as a corruption of *guttur.*   *Cretin* is, in like manner, supposed
to be a corruption of *Chretien* (Christian) a name imposed by a very
natural association ; as a happy prejudice appears to have prevailed
among the uncivilized of all nations in favour of such and other ideots ;
a prejudice founded on the belief that they must be peculiarly the object
of divine favour, whose natural constitution rendered them incapable
of committing these transgressions which lead to its forfeiture, and to
avoid which altogether, is uniformly found to be beyond the feeble
powers of rational and more perfect humanity.

citing cause. A case is related by Mons. Brun, where on the restoration of these, the tumour disappeared.*

When the disease is endemial, it is most generally observed to be hereditary—When not hereditary, it generally makes its appearance about the age of seven or eight. There is a great variety in the size and form of goitres, the disease affecting, in some cases one, in others two, and sometimes the three portions of the thyroid gland. It sometimes attains the size of seven or eight pounds. The consistence of the tumour also varies in character, from that which is most generally met with, and which seems to be a simple enlargement of the thyroid gland, moveable and not adherent to any of the neighbouring parts, to that of a stony hardness. Goitre, in some instances, is supposed to be connected with a scrophulous constitution, and I have observed a few cases where the lymphatic glands about the angle of the jaw were enlarged at the same time with the thyroid. In general, goitres, I believe, produce no bad effects, though certainly in some cases they have produced suffocation from pressure on the Trachæa. When large, they also give a tendency to apoplexy.

* Thesis Sur Bronchocele, Paris 1815.

In a large proportion of cases burnt sponge
(which is given in wine), with friction on the
tumour, is said to have frequently a powerful
effect in dissipating it. In many cases the
effects produced by this medicine on the tumour
are only temporary, in a still greater number,
probably, it fails altogether. The disease is said
to be more difficult of cure when affecting the
middle lobe of the gland. In some cases, the
removal of the swelling is followed by marasmus,
occasionally attended with fever. In one case,
in which the medical attendant advised the
patient not to attempt its removal, marasmus succeeded in such a degree as to endanger life, and
his health and goitre returned together. How
far the direct action of the burnt sponge contri-
buted to produce any of these symptoms, 1 am
not prepared to say : in whatever form it is
taken, it is believed more successful when allowed
to dissolve slowly in the mouth.—The occasional
use of purgatives also aids its effects, and of
course the suppression of any discharge, or any
other remediable state of the system, that may
appear connected with the formation or increase
of the goitre, will be attended to. Friction over
the swelling, and keeping the neck warm, will
also assist in dispersing it, and change to a more
dry and airy situation will prevent a relapse.

By such means as these, Dr. Foderé himself was cured of a goitre which he had till he was fifteen years old.

Dr. Wylie of Petersburg is said to use, with good effect, friction with an ointment composed of half an ounce of litharge ointment, a drachm of calomel, and ten grains of tartrite of antimony.

Where these means have failed, which is very often the case, various chirurgical plans of removing the tumour have been tried, independently of simple extirpation. Mr. Major thinks there are cases where it might be removed by ligature, and mentioned one case to me where this succeeded. He tried it himself in another, but, from the neglect of the attendant, he lost his patient by hæmorrhage, or rather by the low fever which followed this. This gentleman met with a case, where, though the external swelling was very small, the patient complained of being on the point of suffocation, and requested the tumour to be removed at all risk. On making an incision down on the gland, he suddenly pushed away the operator's hand, and got up exclaiming he was perfectly relieved. A membranous fascia had been divided, which allowed the swelling to project externally, and removed the pressure from the trachæa. Such an operation in other cases might be kept in view, as, perhaps, affording the means of saving the patient from threatened suffocation.

A Seton passed through the tumour, is another practice which has been tried by some of the continental surgeons for the removal of goitre, and has succeeded in some cases; but I am informed, after a fair trial of this plan, by Mr. Qardre, a Surgeon of high reputation at Naples, who was very sanguine from the result of his first cases, it has been given up; as several of his patients have died from the fever following the operation.* Indeed, I believe that in the present state of our knowledge, or rather ignorance, of the nature, and causes of this disease and of the functions of the gland which it affects, little should be attempted, in the generality of cases, but change of scene when the complaint appears to be connected with peculiarity in the locality or climate.

I have now brought to a conclusion the observations I had to make concerning the climates of those situations most frequented by consumptive patients in France and Italy, and, I hope I have put medical men in possession of

* An account of these operations has been published since this was written in the last vol. of the Medico-Chirurg. Transactions.

some information that may at least assist them in making up their minds on the propriety of sending their patients to these climates, and also, on the selection of the most advantageous place of residence. I think I have shewn that little is to be expected from sending them to the South of France or Nice; without having adduced equal evidence on Naples, I am, nevertheless, of opinion, that it is as bad as either. The choice, then, as far as my observation goes, appears to lie between Rome and Pisa. Future observations must determine which of these deserves the preference ; and, perhaps, whether the benefit to be derived from a winter's residence at either, is sufficient to repay the inconveniences attending so long a journey, when the disease has made any progress.

In drawing up these observations, where I have ventured to give my own opinion on the effects of climate, I hope it has been with that diffidence which the difficulty of the subject requires. Where circumstances admitted, I have been careful to state the grounds upon which my opinion was founded, the better to enable the reader to form his own judgment on the credit it deserved.

There are two principal circumstances in considering a place of residence in a medical point of view—First, the general nature of its climate, and, secondly, the effects of this on disease. The first may be ascertained without much difficulty, The second is attended with very considerable difficulty,—requires much cautious observation, and the experience of a far greater number of cases than generally come under the observation of any individual. It is on this point that much information is still wanted, as it is by experience alone that the question of the propriety or impropriety of sending our consumptive patients abroad, can finally and for ever be set at rest. To repeat what I have before observed—I am not without hopes that these remarks may have at least this utility, namely, of inducing the medical men who have visited, and who are annually visiting these climates to make their observations public. I shall only further add, that if from future observation I find that any opinion I have given in these pages has been too hastily formed, or is contradicted by further experience, I shall take the earliest opportunity of making it known, as my only object is to ascertain the truth.

To sum up in a few words the opinion I have formed from all the observations I have been enabled to make on the effects of climate in pulmonary consumption—It appears to me,

then, that the change of our English climate
for a residence in the milder ones of the south
of Europe, is much more beneficial as a preventive of the disease, than, I fear, it will ever be
found as a means of cure of it when formed. In
the young and growing members of delicate,
scrophulous and consumptive families, however,
continued for some winters during that age
when the body is attaining its full growth, and
when catarrhal affections are attended with the
greatest danger, it may have great influence in
checking the tendency to hereditary disease.
Even when tubercles already exist in the lungs
in a state of irritation, a residence for some
years in a mild temperature, together with the
adoption of a proper regimen, may be the means
of allaying the irritation, and consequently of
preventing the suppuration of these tubercles.
By a little future attention in guarding against
the known exciting causes of inflammation,
these may long, and perhaps for life, remain in
a state of quiescence. By such measures, and
a strict adherence to the other means most
proper for strengthening the constitution, and
by acquiring habits calculated to inure the body
to the cold and inequalities of its native climate,
(among which I consider the habitual use of the

cold bath as pre-eminent) I have no doubt that many lives might be saved.* When, however, suppuration has actually taken place in the substance of the tubercles, my opinion is, that little or no benefit is to be expected from a change of climate in the cure of the disease; and further, that by the great and numerous inconveniences and discomforts of so long a journey, the fatal termination of it is more frequently accelerated than protracted. That this is very frequently the case in the very advanced stages of the disease, such as I have frequently met with on the Continent shortly after their arrival from England, I have no manner of doubt.

There is still a circumstance connected with the object of this essay on which I must beg leave to say a few words, I mean the state in which many consumptive patients are sent abroad. In the remarks I am about to make I beg explicity to state that I have no intention to

* See Author's Thesis " De Frigoris Effectibus in Corpus vivum," published at Edinburgh, in 1817, for detailed observations on the influence of the cold bath in strengthening the body and enabling it to bear cold.

It is the opinion of some medical men that cold alone is sufficient for the production of tubercles in the lungs, and certainly it is a common cause of inflammation and suppuration of them—Dr. Broussais's observations of the comparative rarity of pulmonary consumptions among the French troops after their entering Italy is deserving of remark.

censure any one. I am aware of the difficult situation in which a medical man is placed when called to decide upon a point where he must often find his information deficient, and where the wisest and best informed may err.

During my residence on the continent I have had frequent occasions to remark with surprize the very advanced stages of the disease in which many of our consumptive patients were sent abroad. This is the more remarkable, as, however medical men may differ about the propriety of sending such patients abroad in the earlier, there surely ought to be no question about its impropriety in the latter stages. For my own part, I have seen enough to convince me that it is not only a very useless, but often a very cruel thing to banish such patients from all the comforts of home, and send them forth to undertake a long journey through a foreign country, deprived probably of all they hold dearest to them, and without those thousand nameless comforts by which the watchful care of friends may cheer even the last period of a hopeless disease. The medical man who reflects on the distresses that such patients must be liable to during such a journey, arrested perhaps in their progress by the increase of some of those symtoms which attend the advanced stages of consumption,—

in very indifferent accommodations, probably, and far from any medical advice in which they can confide,—will surely long hesitate ere he condemns the fated victim of this remorseless malady to the additional evils of expatriation: And his motives for hesitation will be increased when he considers how often the unfortunate patient sinks a prey to his disease long before he reaches the place of his destination; or, at best, arrives at it in a much worse condition than when he left England, and doomed, shortly, to add another name to the long and melancholy list of his countrymen that have sought out, with pain and suffering, a distant country, only to gain in it an untimely grave!

In the foregoing observations I have perhaps viewed matters in the worst light; but it is the duty of the physician in giving his advice in such cases, to keep in mind the possibility of such occurrences. This is in a more peculiar manner necessary with females, upon whom all the inconveniences of travelling fall with double severity. To those acquainted with travelling in many parts of the Continent, it is not necessary to enter into particulars on this subject; and those who are not, may rest assured of the accuracy of what I state. That I do not exaggerate, and to show that these opinions were formed from actual

observation. I shall state a few of the cases that
came to my own knowledge in one season.

The first was that of a young man who was
carried from Bordeaux the greater part of the
way on men's shoulders. When he reached Aix,
about eighteen miles from Marseilles, he could
be carried no farther. An English physician,
then at the latter place, was immediately sent
for and arrived in time to see him expire! This is
an extreme case, I grant, but it shews how far
the eager hopes of relations will lead them in such
cases, if not informed of their error. Several
other patients came to my knowledge, the same
season, who never reached their destination.
One died at Paris ; another at Tours ; and a third
on the way down the Rhine.*   One young man
reached Hieres with difficulty, and lived ten
days. One lady left England in December to
linger a few weeks under the cloudless skies of
Nice, where she died in the end of February or
beginning of March. What a recompence for such
a journey over the roads of France, and with the
discomforts a lady must encounter in many of
the smaller inns of that country!

---

* It is no unfrequent thing to observe in the newspaper obituary
reports, the deaths of persons at Paris, or some other place " on his
way to the South of France." This is some consumptive patient sent
abroad probably in the last stage of his disease to have the short career
he had to run shortened, and to die long ere he reached the place of
his destination.

Should what I have just related reach the eye of the relations of any of the individuals whose cases I have alluded to, I intreat them not to think I wish to excite a painful recollection. I have sympathized with the affliction of several of them at the events I have mentioned, and surely they will not be adverse to my making the only use of this melancholy experience that it is susceptible of, namely, to prevent others of their country-men from suffering under similar circumstances. It is from such experience being generally lost to all but the sufferers that I have had to record so many instances of the kind here. It is surely the duty of the Physician to caution the relations of the patient from indulging hopes which he knows are soon to be cruelly disappointed, and that, perhaps, under circumstances which greatly aggravate the calamity.

I admit that it is natural for the relations to to feel a satisfaction in doing every thing that presents even a prospect of relief, or of delaying as long as possible the event which cannot be prevented ; and change of climate is often considered in this light—as the *anceps remedium :* But the relations should surely be informed in such cases that the period had passed when a change of climate presented any prospect of advantage, and that by dragging the unfortunate victim of this terrible disease to the distant shores of the Mediterranean, they are hurrying on the occurrence of the event they vainly hope to keep off. Patients in the *advanced* stage of consumption would act more wisely in trying the effects of the milder parts of our own island, and, where that fails, they will pass the winter-months with more comfort, and I believe with as much prospect of advantage, in rooms kept at a graduated temperature, amidst friends and all the comforts of home, as they would do by a residence at most of the places frequented abroad,—still taking into the account the inconveniences of the journey thither. This remark is more particularly applicable to females, whose habits are much more congenial to such a mode of living, and who suffer in a far greater degree all the inconveniences and hardships of travelling.

END OF PART FIRST.

Q

PART SECOND.

NOTES

ON THE

Present State of Medicine,

AND

Medical Practice,

IN SOME OF THE

HOSPITALS AND MEDICAL SCHOOLS

OF

FRANCE and ITALY.

—————— Differe quoque, pro natura locorum, genera Medicinæ, et aliud opus esse Romæ, aliud in Ægypto, aliud in Gallia. CELSUS.

PART SECOND.

ON HOSPITALS AND MEDICAL SCHOOLS.

IN submitting the observations contained in this part of the work to Medical
Men, I feel still stronger misgivings than in
that which relates to climate.

My short residence at several of the medical
Schools, of which I have ventured to speak,
may expose me to the imputation of presump-
tion, in attempting to give any account of them.
I am, nevertheless, not without the hope that
the English medical reader will find some information in the following pages, which, if not
very useful, will, at least, be interesting from
the deficiency of knowledge that at this moment exists in England concerning several of
those places ; and thus may feel himself repaid
for the trouble of perusing them. I cannot
certainly flatter myself that my observations
will be received in the favourable manner
which the partiality of some of my medical
friends, in whose judgment I have the highest
confidence, and whose friendship is an honour

to me, would induce me to believe; and I
shall be more than satisfied, if they obtain the
humbler estimation which I have above ventured to claim for them.   The only merit I can
pretend to, is that of recording faithfully, and
unbiassed by any thing, what I observed, ob-
truding my own opinions as seldom as possible.

PARIS.

The following notes on the Hospitals of Paris, as well as the others to be submitted to the reader, were taken merely for my own information without the smallest intention of publication. The only hope I have of their being well received, is, that, as far as I know, they contain the only remarks published on the present state of the medical practice of these hospitals, and that therefore, imperfect as they are, they are better than none.*

All the hospitals of Paris are under the direction of a general administration, and from the office of this board, where medical men attend during a certain part of the day to examine them, patients are sent to the different hospitals.† This plan may be attended with some inconvenience to the patients, but has not a few advantages for the practice of medicine.

* From Mr. Cross's excellent work on the medical school of Paris I derived much information, and to it I beg leave to refer the reader for an account of these schools and of the state of surgery in Paris,

† Accidents and urgent cases are received directly without this form.

Through means of this arrangement the physician of any hospital, whose attention is turned more particularly to any disease or class of diseases, by application to the office of central administration, may have such diseases sent to his own hospital. Thus a much greater number of cases of the disease, which is the object of his particular enquiry, is brought under his observation in a given time (an object of no small importance) than could otherwise, or might indeed ever have been. To this plan, perhaps we owe, in a great measure, the excellent works of Corvisart and Bayle, who were both physicians of **La Charité**, which is now, indeed, almost entirely set apart for chronic cases.* To the same circumstance more lately are we indebted for the excellent work of Dr. Laennec on the diagnosis of the diseases of the chest.

All the hospitals are also supplied with their medicines from a general Pharmacy; the most simple remedies only being prepared at the hospitals themselves. In this department every thing seems to be conducted with the

---

* Both these men have fallen victims to the disease the nature of which they have so well elucidated. Bayle died of consumption, and Corvisart, I am told, is sinking under an organic disease of the heart.

greatest care. The chemical and pharmaceutical laboratories are commodious, and the medicines are prepared with the utmost exactitude. A course of lectures, also, is given every winter on pharmaceutical chemistry.

In general the hospitals of Paris are clean and in good order, and for this they are not a little indebted to a class of attendants which we do not possess in our hospitals, the *sœurs de la Charité*, a religious order of women, who, from principles of religion alone, devote themselves to the care of the sick ; nursing them with a kindness and attention rarely met with in the common nurse, and, at the same time, watching over all the interests of the hospital, and even frequently supplying the most menial offices. These women are always particularly clean and neatly dressed, and whoever has visited these hospitals and beheld their respectable appearance, and the zeal and kindly attention with which they watch over their sick, will be ready to exclaim with Frank—" oh ! se vi fossero in tutti ! Il servigio agli ammalati prestato per solo stimolo di religione e d umanità, quanto non é preferibile al mercenario !"

It is indeed much to be wished that women influenced by such motives should be found in every country to watch over the poor sick.

R

With all the advantages which the medical
men in Paris have in their hospital practice, it is
not a little surprizing that the profession there,
—I always refer to the medical part,—should
hold no higher character than it now does, when
compared to the state of medicine in England,
and, I would add, to the better parts of Italy.
This in a great measure must arise from the medical men not taking advantage of the opportunities
afforded them.   Generally speaking, the physicians in the hospitals of Paris (as appears to me)
have too many patients to attend.   Though it
was summer when I last visited them, and
there were extremely few fevers or acute diseases, yet Dr. Fouquier of La Charité had 104
patients under his own charge with one assistant
only.   Dr. Recamier of the Hotel Dieu had 110,
and the physicians of St. Louis had a still
larger proportion.

The fatal cases are generally examined after
death.   Dr. Fouquier told me that for twelve
years, that he had been physician to La Charité,
no patient had died without being examined.

It is allowed that post mortem examinations,
when properly conducted, form one of the principal means of enabling the physician to acquire
an intimate knowledge of the nature of disease,
and to lead to those principles which are to

guide him in the treatment of it. But the knowledge derived from these examinations, with
whatever care they may be performed, when
taken by itself is but of little real utility. If the
previous history of the disease be not accurately
known, little is to be expected from them ; and
it is a deficiency of this knowledge that appears
to me the principal circumstance which has rendered these examinations at the hospitals of
Paris of so little real value. I have attended not
a few of these examinations, and seen the surprize excited at some appearances, which—had
the morbid phenomena during the course of the
disease been carefully observed—must have been
known, at least, if they could not have been
remedied ; and I have also had occasion to
remark the difference that sometimes occurred
between the physician and assistants with respect to previous symptoms. All this convinced me how truly useful these researches
might have proved but for the want of information relative to the history and progress of the
disease. This circumstance, however, certainly
cannot be sufficiently attended to, where the
physician has so many patients under his care.
I was also convinced by this that clinical
wards, where a few cases are thoroughly attended to, and where the symptoms during life,

and the appearances after death reflect light on
each other, are infinitely better adapted to the
purposes of professional improvement. I must
remark, however, that I speak rather of what
might have been done than of what has been
done. Corvisart and Bayle, and Laennec more
lately, have done much to elucidate the diseases
of the chest; and Bayle was, unfortunately for
the profession, carried off when prosecuting his
researches on the diseases of the other viscera.

If the examinations after death have not
been very well conducted in other diseases, we
fear they have in fevers been almost altogether
neglected in France, as well as in our own country, until very lately. " Nous ne voulons pas
dire (says a late writer) que, jusques aux travaux
de Bayle et de ses condisciples, on s'était ab-
stenu de rechercher le siége des maladies; ce-
pendant on doit avouer que dans les fiévres cette
recherche avait été négligée ou faite avec peu
de pérsevérance, ou même avec prévention."*

In fevers, the neglect of such researches, or
the carelessness with which they are made, is
much to be regretted; as a knowledge of fever
stands in the same relation to physic as that of

---

* Considérations Sur l'état de la médicine en France, depuis la
révolution jusqu'a nos jours. Par J. B. Regnault Chevalier de l'ordre
de St Michel, &c. &c. &c. Paris, 1819—p. 21.

inflammation does to surgery; for, if there is no
surgical disease of which inflammation does not,
or is not liable to form a part,—what disease
comes under the care of the physician in which
fever is not liable to occur at one period or other
during its progress, and even to become the
prominent feature? If the late researches on this
subject are found correct, these two diseases
which have so long been considered generally as
independent of each other, will be viewed but
as cause and effect, and the treatment assume
a precision hitherto unknown. It is by examinations like those lately instituted by Dr.
Broussais of Paris, and by the physicians of our
own country, (particularly in Ireland, where,
unfortunately, too many opportunities of improving our knowledge in this way have lately occurred,) that we can expect medicine to arrive
at the degree of perfection hinted at in the following words of the French author already
quoted: " La pratique et la théorie se prêteront
un mutuel secours; l'experience mieux con-
sultée sera mieux comprise; le langage medical
ne sera plus en opposition avec la conduite
des praticiens, et tous les doutes sur la certi-
tude de la médecine provoqués par le scan-
dale de la discordance des sectes, seront
dissipés.'

LA CHARITE.

The wards of this Hospital are large, clean, well lighted, and well ventilated. Dr. Fouquier is the principal physician, and gives lectures on the practice of medicine, and also clinical lectures on the cases of his own patients. At the time I saw this hospital, the diseases were, as they generally are, almost all chronic ;—a great proportion of them being pulmonary consumption. There were, however, several interesting cases, and the following, among others, particularly attracted my attention, and shews strongly the good effects of venesection in a dropsical affection apparently depending on disease of the heart.

It was that of a soldier, a stout looking man, about fifty : a few days previous to his coming into the hospital, he had lost about forty ounces of blood from the urethra, in consequence of endeavours to force a bougie through a stricture ; the bleeding was stopt, after some time, by the application of cold water. A few days after this, he complained of dyspnœa accompanied with cough and violent palpitation of the heart. General œdema shewed itself, particularly on the right side,

and the dyspnœa and cough increased; his
pulse continuing full, though not hard, he was
bled three times to about ten ounces each
time, in the course of a few days; each bleeding
afforded relief, particularly the last, after which
the œdema began to diminish and soon disappeared almost entirely, while the palpitation
continued. The disease of the heart was considered the sole cause of the dropsical affection,
—organic diseases of this organ often existing
for a considerable time, without exhibiting any
evident symptoms, till the application of cold,
or some other cause deranges the balance of the
circulation:—in the present instance, the loss
of blood might have had this effect, and perhaps, the application of cold, necessary to stop
it might have assisted. The case appeared to
me worthy of remark as a dropsical affection
succeeding the loss of a considerable quantity
of blood cured by the judicious abstraction of
more blood.

Another case which attracted my attention,
from its novelty, was that of a young woman
about twenty-two years of age using the Nux
Vomica for a paralytic affection of the lower extremities. She had been using it for a month,
and the dose had been augmented, during that
time, to eighteen grains of the alcoholic extract.
This quantity she had taken for two days before

I saw her. The first day she only complained
of head ache, for which sinapisms (a very favourite remedy in France) were applied to the
feet, and she took the same dose next day.
On the following night she was attacked by
violent convulsions, and the next morning I
found her apparently suffering much pain which
she referred chiefly to the region of the stomach,
the lower extremities, and abdominal muscles.
These spasmodic pains—sometimes amounting
to a degree of tetanus—appeared to me to
affect the diaphragm. Her pulse was frequent,
the skin hot, but moist. In about ten hours
the convulsions left her, and she became easy ;
though the lower extremities continued rigid,
and affected with occasional spasmodic twitches.
Nothing was done for these spasms, which
were considered of little consequence. The
medicine was laid aside for one day only and
then recommenced in a dose of ten grains,
which I found in the course of a few days
after augmented to fourteen. Dr. Fouquier
thought the application of the sinapisms had
some share in exciting these tetanic symptoms
in the present instance.

I found four other paralytic patients in
Dr. Fouquier's wards using the nux vomica;
in two cases with apparent advantage. Dr.
Fouquier was the first physician to employ this

powerful drug in paralysis, and he was led to do so from observing that the animals killed by it, in the experiments of Mr. Magendie and others, died of tetanus. Elated with his first success he introduced his new remedy with the highest encomiums : "Je viens"—he says in the first part of his memoir on the subject, "annoncer aux medicins un specific nouveau"; and, after relating sixteen cases, (which are far, by the way, from supporting these extravagant praises), he adds,—" I doubt not but it will, at least, generally obtain the confidence, which its early success appears to claim for it; if indeed we are not to expect that the nux vomica shall prove a more infalible remedy in paralysis than the bark in intermitted fevers and mercury in syphilis."*

Like all other remedies introduced with extravagant praises, which the experience of others was far from finding fulfilled, the nux vomica appears about to sink into unmerited neglect in the cure of paralytic disorders. The cases related however by Dr. Fouquier and others, and the singular property of this medicine, when given in moderate doses, of affecting only the paralysed muscles are suffi-

See his " Memoir Sur l'usage do la noix vomique dans le traitement de la Paralysie" p. 16.

S

cient to give it a claim to the attention of medical men, in a disease which too often baffles
every effort of medicine. The effects produced
on the paralytic muscles are various ; generally
rigidity and occasional spasms are the symptoms observed ; in other cases—pains—a sensation of heat—of itching or painful pricking,
sometimes a sense of heat in the stomach : or
of lightness and oppression about the chest :
the appetite generally increases, and the bowels
become constipated during its use. Dr. F.
gives it in the form of alcoholic extract (which
is double the strength of the nux vomica),
in doses of two grains, repeated through the
day ; beginning with one or two, and gradually
increasing it to eight or ten, according to the
effect produced. It generally shews its influence on the parts affected half an hour after
it is taken. When an over dose is given, the
spasms are often very violent, but seem little
liable to attack the diaphragm, which Dr. F.
thinks the reason why they have never killed.
This opinion, however, from the case I have
related appears to me very doubtful ; and
besides, it has frequently been fatal since Dr.
F. wrote his paper.

Dr. Fouquier does not state clearly in his
memoir what are the cases most benefited by

this medicine. It appears to promise most benefit in cases of paraphlegia, or of partial parralysis from rheumatism, cold, &c. &c., and he rather cautions against its use in paralysis following apoplexy, and that where the mental powers are much affected. Among the paralytic patients of La Charité, however, he seemed to use it indiscriminately in all cases. His first expectations appear to have considerably abated, but he informed me that he still thought it the best remedy; although, in some cases, it was useless, and in others might do harm. I believe he is about to publish a new edition of his memoir, in which he means to detail the cases of the latter description—a very necessary measure, as well for his own character, as the cause of science.*

Dr. Esquirol related two fatal cases to me, arising from the use of this medicine. One was that of a woman who had been taking the extract in the increased dose of 18 grains. She had taken this dose *two* days; after the

---

* The active principle upon which the poisonous qualities of the nux vomica depends, was discovered by the French chemists to be a peculiar alkaline substance, and it was named *Vauqueline* after the celebrated chemist of that name; but the academy, indignant that one of its members—" renommé autant par sa douçeur et sa modestie que par ses grands talents, portât le nom d' un substance aussi deletere", changed it to *Strychnie !*

second dose on the second day, she was
seized with convulsions, which ended in death.
On examination, the stomach and bowels
were found in a state of inflammation, and the
vessels of the brain turgid. The other was a
female patient not paralytic:—she took five
grains at once (a second dose, namely, which
was intended for another patient), and expired
after a few convulsions. At one of my visits to
the hospital Saint Louis I was told they had just
been examining a patient who had died from
inflammation of the stomach and bowels produced by this drug. The patient was a negro
servant who had hemiplegia remaining after
a fit of apoplexy. He had taken the extract
of the nux vomica for about ten weeks, and
for the last two weeks, five grains twice a day,
the only effect of it being to produce pains of
the affected parts. At this time he complained
of pain of stomach, and the medicine was
laid aside, but too late;—all the symptoms of
inflammation of the stomach and bowels soon
appeared, and resisted the usual medicines.
On examination after death, the stomach and
intestines were found in an inflamed state, and
several gangrenous spots on the former viscus.
No diseased appearance whatever was observed
in the brain of this patient, nor in those of

three women who died in the Hotel Dieu during
the use of the nux vomica ;—but two of the
latter exhibited evident marks of inflammation
of the stomach.* I met with another case in
some of the French Journals (which I cannot at
this moment recall to my memory) where the
patient died from an enema of a solution of the
nux vomica.

These cases are in opposition to Orfila's
opinion drawn from his experiments with nux
vomica on brutes ; and I may remark that such
experiments are in this instance, as in many
others, very unsatisfactory. It were indeed to
be wished that our physiological experimenters
were a little more cautious in drawing their
conclusions on the effects of medicines on the
human species from those produced on the
mutilated and tortured animals that are the
subjects of their experiments.

I do not mention those fatal cases with a
view of preventing the employment of this
very active medicine, but to show that circum-
spection is necessary in its exhibition. Attention is the more necessary, as, in the above
cases, the violent symptoms are supposed to
have come on without any previous warning.

* Memoir.

I cannot help thinking, however, that if close attention had been paid, (at least in some of the cases) some premonitory signs might have been observed.—The head ache in the first case I have mentioned, occurring in Dr. Fouquier's ward, may perhaps have been some indication. In one case which I saw in these wards, a sensation of heat and uneasiness about the stomach, induced Dr. F., very properly, to suspend the use of the medicine.—This interruption was necessary in several others related in his memoir; and, from the instances I have stated, all unusual feelings about the stomach should be carefully attended to, as should all other symptoms, during the use of so active a medicine. In one case, its use required to be suspended from its remarkable effects upon the brain.

Certain constitutions are more susceptible of the action of this medicine than others. In one case related by Dr. F., slight convulsions were excited by four grains of the nux vomica; yet by cautiously augmenting it, it was carried to fifty-six grains. It would probably be a safe practice during the exhibition of such active medicines (in the solid form) to give them only on alternate days, when they may have been raised to a pretty large dose. We know that the stomach is not at all times in an equally

active state, and that morsels of food of difficult
digestion have been found to remain for a very
long time undissolved in this viscus. It is not
therefore improbable that part, or even the
whole of the medicine, (enveloped, perhaps, in
the indigested food,) may remain for many hours
undissolved ; and that the revived activity of the
stomach about the time of a new dose being given,
may subject the patient to the action of a much
greater quantity than was intended. The external
use of this remedy, as far as I know, has not been
tried.

ST. LOUIS.

This is a very large hospital capable of containing about one thousand patients. It is well situated on a rising ground in the suburbs, and the air is considered so pure that chronic cases are occasionally sent to it from other hospitals. It is the great hospital for cutaneous diseases, and contained during my visits three hundred and fifty such cases, independently of patients affected with psora. To this establishment there are attached four physicians, two surgeons, nine Eleves Internes, and sixteen Eleves Externes.* The wards are generally large, commodious, clean and well ventilated.

* The eleves internes are young men who reside in the hospital as assistants to the physicians and surgeons. After undergoing an examination by concours the student is admitted as an eleve externe, and is employed as a dresser in the surgical wards, and assists the eleve interne in keeping the cases of the patients &c. in the medical department of the hospital. After serving about two years in this capacity they are eligible for the situation of eleve interne. The candidates are numerous and are subjected to another examination. From fifteen to twenty vacancies generally occur every year in the Paris hospitals and for these there are often a hundred and thirty candidates. They frequently remain in this situation for four years and may change their hospital every year, by which they have a more extensive and varied field presented to their observation than the student of most countries. I found many of them extremely intelligent.

In an hospital for the cure of cutaneous diseases the baths form an important part of the establishment. Those of St. Louis are on a very large scale. The common baths, and those for the application of alkaline and other solutions, amounting in all to seventy, are disposed in two large rooms. The general vapour-bath consists of a small room with a flight of steps occupying one side for the patients to sit upon. The vapour flows through an opening in the floor, and the patients regulate the degree of temperature themselves by ringing a small bell, which directs the man who has the charge of admitting it. From twenty to thirty patients may take this bath at the same time. On each side of this is a dressing room kept at a proper temperature. In an adjoining small room are a shower bath, a single vapour-bath, and a partial vapour-bath, the vapour being applied by means of a tube, the orifice of which may be diminished or augmented at pleasure. In another part of the hospital is the sulphur vapour-bath, which can contain twelve patients at once. There is also a single bath of this kind and another for partial fumigations, by which the fumes of mercury, or other substances, may be applied to the face or other parts, without being inhaled during respiration. These baths are appropriated to the use of the male and female

T

patients on alternate days. The success obtained
in the treatment of cutaneous diseases by the
means adopted in this hospital, does not appear
greater than elsewhere.

I observed an extraordinary case of ichthyosis
in a boy about ten years old, where the whole
surface was covered with coarse thick scales.
The cases of tinea capitis are here committed to
the charge of Friar Mahon, who has been making
use of a secret remedy in the cure of this disease,
which rarely fails of success, but is often very
tedious in producing a cure. One of the medical
men of this hospital was trying the effects of oxide
of gold, so strenuously recommended by Dr.
Chrestien, of Montpelier, in syphilis. Some fatal
cases, I was told, had occurred in Paris from the
use of this medicine, inflammation in the stomach,
being the effect which led to the fatal termination.

MAISON DES ENFANS MALADES.

This hospital interested me much; it was the first I had seen entirely appropriated to children, and the establishment altogether appeared well conducted and in excellent order. The site is particularly well chosen, being a rising ground in the suburbs of the city; it contains nearly six hundred patients, and has sufficient space for the exercise of the little convalescents. The general plan of this hospital appears very good, though I perfectly agree with Mr. Cross that very little advantage is to be expected from huddling together, in one ward, a crowd of scrophulous children. Indeed this seems to have operated so strongly on the minds of the medical attendants that these poor creatures appear to be left to themselves,—this department of the hospital being in by far the worst condition. It is placed in one corner of the inclosure entirely separated from the other buildings. Some vapour baths were erecting for their use, and from the judicious administration of these I believe much benefit might be derived in many cases of scrophula.*

* For some account of the economy of this hospital and other remarks on the surgical practice, I beg leave to refer the reader to Mr. Cross's work, which, on this, as on every other occasion, where I had an opportunity of comparing it, I found correct.

The only establishment of this kind, probably, that could prove really useful for this unfortunate class of young patients, would be one situated in a healthy part of the country, and which should be considered rather as preventive of this dreadful disease than curative of it. Scrophulous children might here be educated, a large proportion of the day being occupied in exercise in the open air, gardening, agriculture, &c. Cold and warm baths ought to form a part of such an Institution, as also an hospital for the cases requiring particular medical attendance, and the medical superintendant of this should direct the economy of the whole establishment. A nourishing diet and bountiful supply of clothing would form two of the most essential requisites. By such an establishment, on a large scale, many of the most useful and ornamental members of society might be preserved who are now lost; it being well known that the finest genius is often connected with the delicate structure of the scrophulous constitution.

But to return to our hospital. All patients who die are examined, and on enquiry 1 was told that pulmonary consumption was a frequent cause of death among these juvenile sufferers; and that even where it was not the immediate cause of death, the lungs exhibited more or less of diseased structure. The number of boys and girls in the hospital is generally nearly equal. The wards are divided into those for acute cases, and those for chronic ones such, as tinea capitis, psora, &c.

In the chronic wards I was rather surprized to find almost every one of the little patients labouring under inflammation of the eyes, many in a very great degree, though generally the eyelids were chiefly affected. Whether the indiscriminate use of towels might not be the means of communicating even this chronic degree of ophthalmia, appears to me a question that at any rate deserves attention. These cases seemed not to attract the observation of their medical attendants, a circumstance which we have daily occasion to remark in the slight, and apparently insignificant affections of the eyes, which, however, too often lay the foundation for future loss of vision, and which, by a little attention in the early stages of the complaint, might have been easily prevented. It is rather surprizing, considering the very great frequency of diseases of the eyes, that there are not more establishments set particularly apart for them. I believe that no one of this nature exists in Paris, or even in all France.

The small-pox wards, I was pleased to find, did not contain a single case; and the medical gentleman who attended me, and who had been paying particular attention to that disease, in-

formed me that they had seen but little of it
during the last twelve months, although all the
poor children labouring under the disease in Paris
are sent to this hospital. In the spring of 1818,
small-pox was very frequent in Paris, and very
fatal; more than half of those admitted into this
hospital sometimes dying.*

Strange to say, the heating, and sudorific plan
was the one adopted at this time in the treatment
of these little patients! All those who died were
examined, and the appearances observed were
inflammation and ulceration of the internal coat
of the intestines, pustular eruptions there, or on
the surface of the peritoneum; and, in three
cases, a false membrane, similar to that of
croup, was found lining the whole alimentary
canal from the œsophagus to the rectum: in these
three cases, the eruption on the surface had
never shown itself distinctly. These morbid
appearances called the attention of the medical
officers to Dr. Broussais's opinions; the cooling
antiphlogistic treatment, with the application of
leeches over the abdomen, was adopted in conse-

* It was epidemic in Edinburgh I find and in various other parts of
the kingdom at the same time. See Dr. Hennen's paper in the 14th vol.
of the Edin. Med. Journal.

The rapidity with which epidemics travel over Europe, so as to
cause their contemporaneous appearance in distant quarters is a subject that might give rise to a great deal of curious speculation.

quence, and the speedy reduction of the mortality soon evinced the superiority of the practice.

The following statement of the proportion of deaths from this disease is interesting on many accounts ; and, taken in conjunction with the circumstance just detailed, cannot fail to make a strong impression on the mind of the English reader.

Small-pox cases admitted into the hospital des Enfans Malades, in 1816, 1817, and 1818 :

		Cured.	Died.	Total.
1816	....	42	53	95
1817	[From Jan. to Aug.]	51	37	88
1818	.. ..	117	102	219
		210	192	402

Whether such an establishment as the one just described could be introduced into England appears to me very questionable, though of its utility there can be little doubt. It may be doubted whether English mothers could be induced to give up their children to the care of strangers ; they certainly would not have, in our hospitals, to consign them to the care of that good sisterhood who supply the place of the most attentive mothers to their little patients. I found fourteen of these nuns employed about this hospital.

As a school for observing the diseases of childhood, under all their various forms, this establishment is invaluable to the medical student of Paris.

HÔPITAL NECKER.

Close to the Hospital I have described is that endowed by the wife of M. Necker the celebrated minister of state. It is a small hospital containing about a hundred and thirty patients; but, from being the one in which the late experiments of Dr. Laennec on the diagnosis of diseases of the thorax were made, I visited it frequently with the view of ascertaining the utility of his method. Dr. Laennec was indisposed, but his colleague Dr. Cayol pointed out to me several cases where the information gained by the application of the *sthenoscope* was useful in ascertaining the nature of the disease. I found, however, that it would require more time than I had to bestow to make myself fully acquainted with the use of this instrument. Nevertheless I observed enough to convince me that much useful information is to be acquired through the medium of this instrument in distinguishing the disease of the different viscera of the thorax.

The instrument used by Doctor Laennec for this purpose is a perforated cylinder of wood about thirteen inches long, the perforation being about four or five lines in diameter; it is

divided into two parts and scooped out at one
of the extremities. When used, one end is
applied to the chest of the patient and the ear of
the physician to the other, and from the peculiar
sound communicated through the medium of the
instrument, while the patient is speaking, or
breathing, or by the pulsation of the heart,
the physician is enabled to ascertain the nature,
and often the extent of the disease more accurately than has hitherto been done by any other
means. Several medical men in Paris, I found,
thought highly of this new method, and the
report of the Institute is very favourable. Dr.
Recamier, in particular, one of the physicians
of the Hotel Dieu, informed me, whilst going
round his wards, that he could accurately dis-
cover the extent of injury in most diseases of the
lungs by means of the cylinder, which he carried constantly in his hand.

It has been asked in reference to Dr. Laennec's discovery, what it will avail us to know
the exact situation of an ulcer in the lungs, or
whether it is a little larger, or smaller than we
believed?—whether we shall be better able to
cure an organic affection of the heart or large
blood vessels, by knowing the particular part
affected? The remark is futile, and has a tendency to check philosophic research. To know

the nature and extent of a disease is surely the
first step in our progress to the adoption of
rational means of cure; and though the diseases particularly alluded to, are, unfortunately,
beyond the known powers of medicine, the profession has not assuredly arrived at that degree
of perfection to entitle us to pronounce that they
will always remain so. But setting aside
other advantages, it must surely be highly
satisfactory to every ingenuous mind to know
the exact nature of the disease under which a
patient labours, even when it is known to be
incurable. How often the mind of the physician
is lost in vague conjecture throughout the whole
progress of some of the diseases alluded to, experience can best tell.

It is also sometimes of much importance to
be able to give an accurate prognosis of a disease which is incurable ; and this can often only
be done by a knowledge of its extent, of which
the symptoms generally relied on, are so often a
fallacious indication. Among the consumptive
cases which I lately met with abroad, I have had
frequent occasion to remark how widely some
of our best practitioners have erred in foretelling
the termination of a disease ; a proof, not of
ignorance, but that the symptoms usually
trusted to are insufficient even to guide the most

experienced in their prognosis. I had lately a case under my charge which excited much interest, where, from the closest attention to all the symptoms, no physician would have been warranted in giving the prognosis which the ultimate result of the case showed to be the correct one. Had I been acquainted with Dr. Laennec's method (not then published) I could have ascertained the extent of disease in the chest which the usual symptoms did not indicate, and could thus, at least, have been enabled to prevent much inconvenience, and perhaps the rise of hopes which were to be soon blighted.

In consultation with some other medical men, I witnessed the case of a Piedmontese at Rome, who was supposed to labour under some extensive organic disease of the heart or aorta. In this case the palpitation at times was extremely violent and the dyspnœa very great. Little had been done before we saw this patient, and the remedies used afterwards had only the effect of mitigating the symptoms for a time. General dropsy soon appeared, and the patient, as frequently happens in such cases, died of apoplexy. On examination after death the only unusual appearance about the heart was a slight enlargement of that organ; the pericardium contained much serum and the chest on both sides was filled with the same fluid, the lungs being greatly compressed. Had the nature of this poor man's disease been known at the beginning, there is no reason to believe that his life might not have been prolonged, perhaps for years.

This was one of those numerous cases where affections of the mind appear to produce not only functional but organic disease of the heart. This man had been reduced by the late political changes, from a captain in the French army to the menial office of a waiter in an hotel, while he was, at the same time, an exile from his native land where his property had been confiscated. The chagrin produced by this reverse of fortune he could never get the better of, and I have no doubt that it was the cause of his disease, since late observations have amply shown that the old and ridiculed idea of dying broken-hearted is often but too true.* The above case shows, at any rate, that we should not rashly re-

* For an eloquent expósition of this pathological fact I refer the reader to Corvisart's excellent work on diseases of the heart. 2d. edit vol. 1. p. 369. I make one short extract: " Les scenes sanglantes de la Revolution, leurs hideux tableaux, le bouleversement des fortunes, les saississemens, les emotions, les chagrines qui en ont eté la suite, ont, dans ces derniers tems, fourni une foule de preuves de l'influence des affections morales sur le developpement des maladies organiques en general, et de celles du cœur en particulier. Combien n'avons nous pas vu, dan les hopitaux des personnes naguere opulentes, alors reduites a la mendicité, desirer une morte prompte, que des lesions organiques du cœur leur apportaient trop lentement a leur gré!

ject any means that may be pointed out of increasing our diagnostic knowledge of such important
diseases ; and if Dr. Laennec's discovery supports
the charater given of it, he has conferred an essential service on his profession and mankind in
general, and deserves their grateful thanks ;—
however the more easy-minded part of the profession may smile at the means he uses.

To give an account of the manner of using
the Sthenoscope does not come within the intention of this Essay, and this is of the less consequence as I have reason to believe a full review
of that and of the other parts of Dr. Laennec's
valuable work will appear in an early number of
Dr. Johnson's Medico-Chirurgical Review.*

In all diseases of the chest much attention is
also paid in Paris to the information to be gained
by means of percussion of that cavity by the hand,
a means of information which is little if at all attended to, I believe, in England. A patient
brought into any of the hospitals of Paris with
any affection of the chest, is as regularly submitted
to this process as the English physician would

---

* An English Physician to whom I gave a Sthenoscope which I
brought from Paris with me, informs me he has already found it useful in the diagnosis of some of the diseases of the heart.

ascertain the state of his pulse ; and the high opinion that is entertained of this as a diagnostic in France cannot be more strongly evinced than in the following encomium bestowed on it by the physician above mentioned, who has necessarily given great attention to the investigation of diseases of the Thoracic viscera : " La percussion de la poitrine, suivant la mèthode de l'ingénieux observateur que je viens de citer (Avenbrugger,) est sans contredit l'une des découvertes les plus précieuses dont la médecine se soit jamais enrichie. Elle a soumis au jugement immédiat des sens plusieurs maladies que l'on ne reconnaissait jusque là' qu'à des signes généraux et équivoques, et en a rendu le diagnostic aussi sûr que facile."*

* De L'auscultation médiate ou Traité du Diagnostic Des Maladies Des Poumons et du cœur &c, par R. T. H. Laennec M. D. Paris, 1819. p. 4.

—

MILITARY HOSPITAL OF VAL DE GRACE.

This is a very extensive hospital, and is interesting, if on no other account, from Dr. Broussais being one of the physicians. This physician, whose new views of disease have lately created a considerable sensation among the medical men of Paris, has had immense experience as physician of the army, and still enjoys an extensive field in the great military hospital of Paris.

He gives public lectures, which are numerously attended. His doctrines appear to me highly deserving of the attention of every medical man. They throw considerable light on the origin of febrile diseases, and, whether we adopt his opinions fully or not, his practice in fever, founded on them, is sanctioned by the authority of the best medical practioners of the present day in England. His manner of investigating diseases is strictly philosophical, and the advantages which he has already shewn to arise from such investigations in the illustration of diseased action, will do more good, I believe, in a country where such apathy exists in the medical practice, than all the medical works published in France for the last hundred years.

Were his doctrines, promulgated through the medium of his works and lectures, to have no other effect than that of exciting a spirit of philosophical enquiry among the rising members of the profession in that country (which they cannot fail to do,) they will be of incalculable benefit.

I found few cases of fever in the Val de Grace; indeed there were very few fever cases in any of the hospitals of Paris during the months of July and August when I was there. Dr. Broussais examines all the patients that die in his hospital, and one of the house surgeons assured me he had never been present at one of these examinations where a greater or less degree of inflammation had not existed in the mucous membrane of the stomach and bowels. This, Dr. Broussais considers the seat of the disease; and his treatment of fever, founded on this view of the cause, consists in the application of leeches to the abdomen, in numbers proportioned to the strength of the patient and severity of the disease. The number of leeches applied varies from twenty-five to sixty. One patient was pointed out to me in the hospital, to whom two hundred had been applied in the course of the fever: he was convalescent. Dr.

x

Broussais does not employ general blood-letting, as he thinks it little useful in inflammation of the mucous membranes. The increased action of the heart and arteries in fever he considers merely symptomatic of the local affection.— Allowing this to be the case, which is more than many will allow, still this increased action must in its turn increase the local affection, and whatever reduces this increased action of the heart and arteries, must have a beneficial influence on the latter. There are many cases, I believe, wherein the local abstraction of blood will not entirely supersede the use of the lancet, but I do think it might, with great advantage, be brought more into the aid of the former in the fevers of Great Britain, than it is.

I am by no means adverse to general bleed- ing in fevers ; I have witnessed and experienced its very beneficial effects on a large scale ; but if the local abstraction of blood is less injurious to the constitution than the general, (which I believe is generally admitted,) and if Dr. Broussais finds the former so beneficial as to render, in his opinion, the latter unnecessary in fever, it is reasonable to believe that local might be brought more into the assistance of general blood-letting than it is, particularly in the young, and in more feeble constitutions.

In dysentery, too, where, if the state of the
vessels of the lining membrane of the intestines
is not admitted to be actual inflammation, it is
at least now allowed by the best practitioners
to require the same treatment; there is every
reason from analogy to believe, that the liberal
application of leeches to the abdomen will be
found highly useful in obviating the necessity of
venæsection, to the same extent that might be
otherwise necessary, and free the minds of many
practitioners from the bugbear debility, which
is so much dreaded after general bleeding—and
that more in dysentery perhaps than in any
other disease.   This is accordingly the practice,
and, according to the published report of his
doctrines, the successful practice of Dr. Broussais in this disease.

Emetics, purgatives, and blisters are con-
demned by Dr. B. in fevers, from their supposed tendency to augment directly, or by
sympathy, the inflammation of the membrane
of the stomach and bowels.   The inflammatory affections of the throat and trachea, in
measles and scarlatina, he treats by the application of leeches, as he does acute rheumatism.   In one of his wards a soldier was pointed
out to me who had lately come into the hospital with acute rheumatism of both knee and

ankle joints, accompanied with the usual symptoms of redness, heat, and swelling.   Sixty
leeches were distributed on these joints, which
bled freely ; next day the patient was free from
pain and the swelling of the joints gone.   Both
thumb joints were afterwards affected in the
same way, and a large number of leeches,
applied to each, removed the disease with the
same rapidity as in the case of the knee and
ankle joints.*   By this prompt abstraction of
blood from the affected parts I was informed
his success in the treatment of acute rheumatism
is very great.†

I shall conclude these cursory remarks on
Dr. Broussais s doctrines and practice by the
following character of him written by the
author of the   *Considerations'* already referred

---

* This practice may be contrasted with that at Marseilles (men
tioned in page 16 of Part First,) in the case of the unfortunate English
sailor who had his swollen joints kept enveloped for months in warm
poultices, as if to prevent the possibility of nature effecting a cure,
which she might have done during the time the poor man was confined in the hospital.

† The only account yet given to the public of Dr. Broussais's new
doctrines is contained in a small work just published by two of his pupils
Drs. Caignou and Quémont, entitled " Leçons du Docteur Broussais sur
" les Phlegmasies gastriques, dites Fievres continues essentielles des
" auteurs, et sur les phlegmasies cutanées aigües," Paris, 1819.

to, and which is deserving of the more notice, as that gentleman seems scarcely to have escaped himself altogether from the trammels of the expectant system. " Ce médecin habile a fait ressortir avec la plus grande force l' importance de la recherche du siége des maladies, l'utilité des antiphlogistiques dans un grand nombre de cas où l' on s'efforcait de les proscrire d' apres des idées purement spéculatives ; il a fait remarquer que dans les fiévres l'inflammation joue un trés-grand rôle, et qu'il importe d'y avoir égard pour le choix des moyens curatifs ; il a fait connoître la maniere dont plusieurs phlegmasies chroniques se manifestent, et les modifications que nécessite dans le traitement la nature des tissus malades: tels sont ses titres incontestables á la célébrité."

SALPETRIERE.

This immense establishment is entirely devoted to females,—the deranged, the epileptic, the aged, and the infirm.

The part allotted to the deranged seems to have been built on no regular plan, but at different periods as occasion required The cells are very badly ventilated. To obviate this fault, in some degree, the upper parts of the walls between the cells have been removed and replaced by gratings. By this means, however, the noisy patient in one cell may disturb many of her more peaceable neighbours. The whole number of insane in this hospital amounted at my visit to 1100, and of these 200 were idiots. In the convalescent ward there were 30 individuals. This ward is at present badly placed, being too near the other parts of the hospital with which it communicates. A new one, however, is about to be built, entirely separated by a wall from the other patients. The greatest mildness in the treatment of the patients is adopted in this hospital. Dr. Esquirol is the physician of that department of Salpêtrière appropriated to the deranged ; and whoever has

the pleasure of examining that establishment
with that gentleman will not fail to be pleased
with the manner in which it is conducted, and
with the attention which is paid to the patients.
A greater proof of this attention need not be
given than that in the eleven years during which
Dr. E has had charge of this institution, two
suicides only have occurred. Those who show
any propensity to commit this act, are placed
in the infirmary, where they are more immediately under the eyes of the attendants. There
are no chains no whips to be met with : " La
France (says this gentleman) donne au monde
civilisé l'exemple de plus de deux mille aliénés
de tout âge, de tout sexe, de tout état, de tout
caractre, dirigés, contenuès et trait és sans
coups et sans chaîne."*

Dr. Esquirol has examined all the Lunatic
Establishments in France, and the description
he gives of a large proportion of them is indeed

---

* See his late excellent Report des Maisons des Aliénés en France.
In my late short visit to England I had much satisfaction, on visiting
Bethlehem hospital with Drs. Monro and Wright, to see the same
mild treatment adopted in that establishment. The whole of the arrangements of this excellent institution reflect much credit on all concerned in it, There is, no doubt, still room for improvement, and there
happily appears in the medical officers the best disposition to effect
what is necessary.

dreadful, and forms a striking contrast with that of Salpêtrière. Dr. E. finds that in France in general, the number of deranged women is greater than that of men. In the southern provinces the proportion of males is greater than that of females, while, in the north, the proportion of females is much greater than that of males. During my visits to this excellent establishment several interesting cases were pointed out to me. One patient from the age of eighteen had paroxysms of mania every spring, for five years ; this last spring in place of her usual paroxysms of delirium she was attacked by intermitting fever, which yielded to the usual medicines and she was now well. He mentioned another singular case of periodical mania where the paroxysm was regularly preceded by all the symptoms of phthisis pulmonalis ; after a week's duration these ceased, leaving only a little hoarseness, and the delirium recommenced. By milk diet he thought he kept off the paroxysms for two years, but they eventually returned.

Another patient kept herself constantly buried in the straw of her bed, and would not admit of any other covering. Dr. E. thought it best to leave her undisturbed, from his experience of two other cases that had occurred to him—one of a woman, who, after a violent paroxysm of mania, lay in the same situation for six months, at the end of which period she got up quite well; the other of a young gentleman in his own private establishment who cut his pailliasse every night and buried himself in the straw : at the end of six weeks he also was well. Speaking of relapses he remarked that he had known many cases where a paroxysm had occurred after bleeding; some cases after a small, in others after a large bleeding.

Dr. E. has no confidence in any remedy for epilepsy. He mentioned a case where a large portion of the stomach was destroyed by the use of the nitrate of silver in that disease. At the Bicêtre I found they were giving a pretty extensive trial in that disease to the application of the actual cautery to the head, and in some cases, I was told, with the apparent effect of prolonging the intermission and rendering the paroxysm less severe. The Bicêtre, which is entirely appropriated to men, forms at once an hospital for the deranged, a house of reception for the poor, and a prison for malefactors, but is inferior in accommodation and arrangement to the Salpêtrière.

HÔPITAL DE CLINIQUE INTERNE.

This Hospital is close to La Charité, and was first established by Corvisart, who selected his patients for it from the latter hospital. It contained twenty four male and fourteen female patients when 1 visited it—all chronic cases. The practice appeared to me particularly inert: Ptisanes pectorales—-Eau gommé—-lavement emollient—&c. were among the most active prescriptions, and few escaped without some one or two of these. Tis sickening to an English physician in visiting the hospitals of Paris to hear nothing but these eternal ptisans ordered for every patient, let the disease be chronic or acute. It may be said they are harmless at any rate, and may satisfy the patient that something is doing. But surely the latter consideration is little necessary in hospital practice, and I am inclined to think that the plan is often worse than harmless, as it operates, in some degree, on the mind of the physician, and leaves an impression that he has done something, when, in truth, he has done nothing. In this way, perhaps it prevents the employment of more active means when they are actually requisite. The details of practice just mentioned must appear in a still more striking light when it is considered that this hospital is one '*de perfectionnement*' for those about to take their degrees in medicine, as that of M. Dubois is for those in surgery.*

The cases of the patients are kept in this hospital, but, as in the other instances where this is done, it is only by the pupils. The physician makes no reports himself, but merely orders the medicines, which are noted down at the time. I was indeed disappointed to find the system of practice in this hospital no better than in the others. In a clinical hospital where accurate reports are not daily given by the physician at the bed-side of the patient, the advan-

---

* In the hospital of M. Dubois there was a singular case of horny excrescence occupying the anterior part of the frontal bone and part of the parietal bones. The skin had a red irritable appearance round the base. From its pressing down upon the forehead, it had disfigu-red the woman's countenance. From the base to the apex, which was about two inches above the integuments of the head, it tapered to a point, and she said she suffered much pain from it. It made its appearance two years before over a cicatrice occasioned by a burn when she was a child. An operation in the early stages of this disease would perhaps have entirely removed this excresence. At Toulon in the spring of 1818 I met with a poor woman, a native of Biscay I think, the whole of whose toes and fingers were converted int bony substances and greatly elongated, like talons. The cuticle on many parts of the body was converted into patches of the same horny nature—This poor woman's appearance indicated bad health, and altogether was very miserable.

tages both to the student and physician are in-
calculably diminished. The whole method of
teaching the practice of medicine in Paris appears to me very bad. The author of the review
already quoted observes with much justice—
" L' enseignement de la mèdeciné-pratique n'est
pas encore ce qu'il devrait être et c'est surtout
dans cette partie de nos institutions qu on doit
espérer un perfectionnement vivement désiré
de tous les bons esprits."

To the other Hospitals of Paris my visits
were less frequent, and I shall not trouble the
reader with any account of them. My object has
not been to give a particular account of hospitals, but to observe any thing remarkable in the
state of the medical practice as far as my time
and opportunities admitted: I sought those hospitals chiefly, where it appeared to me this was
most likely to be attained. I fear the few observations I have made will appear very unsatisfactory, but, in truth, I did not find much worthy of remark beyond what I have stated. The
diseases in all the hospitals were mostly chronic,
but, even making allowance for that, the practice in general appeared to me very inert and
very little varied. The young English physician, however, who is well instructed in the

practice of his own country, and who can attend for a few months the Parisian hospitals, will not fail, from the immense field laid open to him, to make many useful observations that may probably benefit himself as well as his countrymen. I shall be glad if the few observations here collected should induce some one better qualified, and with greater command of time, to do justice to the subject. He may be assured that he will meet with ready access to all the medical establishments, and due attention from all the medical officers. It gives me pleasure to bear witness to their great willingness to point out whatever is most worthy of remark, and, in short, to communicate every information that is likely to be either useful or desirable.

I shall conclude this brief view of the practice of some of the Parisian hospitals by a short statement of the proportion of deaths in these during a period of ten years, from (1804 to 1814) extracted from a work, entitled " Rapport fait au conseil General des Hospices par un de ses membres sur l' etat des Hopitaux, &c."

Hotel Dieu.

Admitted during the ten years 101,595
Remaining in the Hospital, 1st Jan. 1804   834

                   Total   102,429
Of this number died in the ten years   20,623
Remained in the Hospital, 31st Dec. 1818   869

The proportion, consequently, of deaths, in this Hospital during the above period was something more than one in five—

One in $4 \frac{93}{100}$ or $4 \frac{28}{100}$ according as we allow or not for the patients remaining at the commencement and termination of the period.

La Charité.

Remaining in the Hospital, Jan. 1804   204
Admitted in the ten years   27,456

                   Total   27,660
Of this number died in the ten years   5,881
Remained 31st Dec 1818   204

Proportional mortality therefore in this Hospital has been about one in $7 \frac{8}{100}$.

L'Hopital des Enfans.

Remaining 1st Jan. 1804   247
Admitted in the ten years   20,667

                   Total   20,914

Of these died 4,688
Remained 31st Dec. 1813 420
    Proportional mortality therefore is one in
4 $\frac{37}{100}$.

Hopital St. Louis.

Remaining 1st Jan. 1804 495
Admitted in ten years 56,934

                   Total 57,429
Of these died in the ten years 2,138
Remained 31st Dec. 1818 1,129
    Proportional mortality therefore is only one
in 26 $\frac{33}{100}$.*

---

* The inferior proportional mortality of St. Louis is accounted for
by the nature of the diseases treated in it, viz. cutaneous eruptions
and other chronic ailments.

LYONS.

Some account of the hospitals and state of medical practice at Lyons may not be an un-acceptable addition to the few preceding re-marks on those of Paris.

HOTEL DIEU. This is the only general hospital in Lyons. It contains nearly twelve hundred beds; and when it is considered that Lyons is a manufacturing town, with a population of nearly one hundred and thirty thousand, and that the hospital is open to all patients that present themselves from whatever place or nation, and to the military, also, stationed in the city, and that its wards are open to all diseases, except syphilis and psora,—its crowded state is not much to be wondered at. The Hotel Dieu, commenced on a magnificent scale, has not been (and certainly ought never to be) finished. Its situation is bad, being confined, low and damp; the Rhone runs close by its front and on all other sides it is closely surrounded by some of the thickest parts of the town. To this low damp situation are attributed the catarrhal affections to which the patients are very subject after surgical

operations, and which renders these less successful than they would be in a more favourable
situation. The plan of this hospital, though in
its present state very incomplete, does not
appear much better chosen than its site. The
wards are too large, and communicate too freely
with each other. There are generally three,
frequently four ranges of beds very close to
each other, and all surrounded with curtains,
which render perfect ventilation difficult.

The principal department for medical cases
is in the form of a Greek cross, the centre being
under a lofty cupola communicating at the top
with the external air. Two of the arms of this
cross are appropriated to male, and the other
two to female patients, without any sepa-
ration between them. The beds are here in
three ranges very close together, and all surrounded by curtains ; yet from the height, the
number of windows both in the side and ends,
and the square openings on a level with the floor
which perforate the wall, and the communication of the central cupola with the external air,
this immense ward, or rather assemblage of
wards, containing between three and four hundred beds, and often nearly twice as many
patients, is kept tolerably well ventilated : I
say twice as many patients—because during

z

winter, when disease is prevalent, it not unfrequently happens that one third of the beds of
this hospital contain two patients each; and
indeed, during my visits in October, 1 observed
this to be the case frequently, in both the medical and surgical departments.

The great surgical ward for men contains upwards of two hundred beds in four ranges, and
this, and the womens' surgical ward, also thickly
planted with beds, were the worst ventilated
parts of the hospital. In the higher parts of the
building are the medical wards for the military,
who are attended by their own medical men.
These wards contained upwards of two hundred
patients, and were not full. There are several
other smaller wards;—one for cases of tinea
capitis,—one for small-pox; in the latter there
were only half a dozen convalescents,—the
cow-pox inoculation being pretty generally
practised at Lyons, though there are usually a
few small-pox cases in the hospital. The latter
disease, 1 was told, had been observed to occur
after the patient had been previously properly
inoculated with cow-pox in a few instances,
but, as usual, such cases have been extremely
mild. A part of the hospital is appropriated to
poor married women during labour. There is
also a department of the hospital for patients that

pay;—one class at the rate of two franks (one shilling and eight pence), and another at twelve franks a day : these last have each a room. Making allowance for the faulty plan of this hospital, and its necessarily crowded state, it was altogether in pretty good condition. The bed-steads are of iron ; the bed curtains white, and, as well as the sheets and other parts of the bed-ding, clean.

The medical establishment of the Hotel Dieu consists of six physicians, two surgeons, a surgeon-major, and an aid-major (who holds his appoint-ment six years, and takes the place of the chief surgeon at the expiration of his time,) and eleven elèves internes who reside in the hospital con-stantly, on a plan similar to those of the Paris hospitals. The inferior class of attendants is ex-tremely numerous, and is truly a burden on the establishment, consisting of about two hundred nuns or sisters, and from forty to fifty friars, besides labourers. These sisters fill the situation of nurses, cooks, assistant apothecaries, &c. and the brothers are chiefly occupied in the offices.*

* I fear some of these are useful only in the same way as I found a kindred class of hangers-on in one of the great Italian hospitals. While going round the wards with one of the physicians I asked him what part of the duty these men performed, and his answer (with a significant gesture) was—" mangiano—bevono—e se divertono"— " They eat, drink, and divert themselves !"

The latter might be dispensed with altogether, and one half of the former would be quite sufficient. Another bad thing is having a public apothecary's shop in the hospital.

A large proportion of the patients in this hospital at the time of my visits were cases of fever, generally very slight, and dependant upon, or connected with, irritation of the mucous coat of the stomach and bowels, forming what the French call ' Fièvre Muqueuse.' Indeed, fevers accompanied with affections of the mucous membranes are the most common diseases of Lyons; which may be accounted for from the low damp situation of the place, and the occupation of a large proportion of the inhabitants in the silk, and other confined and sedentary manufactures.

Lyons is mostly built on a plain, the Rhone washing one side of it, and the Soane passing through the other half; the rivers meeting about a mile below the town. The streets are also very narrow and tortuous and the houses high, which circumstances add to the natural dampness of the situation, and prevent free ventilation. During the winter months fogs are also very frequent.

Among such occupations, and in such a climate, scrophulous affections, as might be foreseen, are frequent. Tabes mesenterica is its most frequent form among children, and pulmonary con-

sumption among those farther advanced in years.
On enquiring into the progress of this disease, I
was told its course was much less rapid than in the
more southern parts of France, as at Marseilles,
—the average duration being about eighteen
months. Goitres, also a frequent attendant on
humidity, are likewise frequent in Lyons.

The practice of the Hotel Dieu, from what
I observed, and was told by one of the physicians,
partakes much of the expectant system, with a
pretty strong bias among some of the physicians
to the Brunonian. The doctrines of Broussais,
however, have had their effect in Lyons. The
inspection of fever cases after death has been
much more attended to, and his observations on
the co-existence of an inflammatory state of the
mucous coat of the stomach and intestines veri-
fied in a considerable proportion of cases ; and
when absent there, marks of local affection have
often been observed in the other viscera, particularly the brain. These examinations have
induced the more liberal and candid part of the
profession here to be more cautious in the exhibition of bark and stimulants, and to look for local
inflammation, as a cause, or at least concomitant,
of those fevers which they before styled nervous,
putrid, malignant, adynamic, &c. and for which
stimulants were considered the only proper reme-

dies. The use of mild diluents, and occasionally the application of leeches, have taken the place of the stimulant system ; but general bleeding is rarely or never had recourse to in fever, being reserved entirely for the more marked phlegmasiæ. A foundation, however, seems to be laid in Lyons, for the destruction of the blind system of Brown, and the little better, but more specious one of Pinel, (which by some of the French medical men is styled *Pinelism.*) and for the adoption of a more close enquiry into the cause and pathology of disease as leading to the only rational method of treatment. The fact, which I have from undoubted authority, that at this moment four fifths of the practitioners of Lyons are Brunonists, will shew how much this was wanted.

Judging from the fever cases which I saw in the hospital, I would say that a less active practice is certainly required than in the fevers that I have generally seen in England ; though, even in those, a more active practice might have been adopted in some cases I conceive, with a considerable advantage. I shall just mention one of these cases of fever that I saw with the physician on his first visit to the subject of it. It occurred in the person of a middle aged woman :—she complained of pricking pains in the epigastric region ; her pulse was tense and rather hard ;

her skin hot, and face rather flushed ; the tongue
covered with a thin white fur—the margins red :
two leeches were ordered to be applied to the anus
—a favourite mode of practice among the French
physicians in several affections, particularly when
the liver is affected, which it was supposed had
been the case with this patient for some time previous to the appearance of fever. This, with
some diluents, was the only thing prescribed.

The average proportion of deaths in this
hospital is something less than one in nine as
will be seen by an extract from an excellent
report of the state of the Hotel Dieu, from June
1812 to June 1813, (since which no report has
been published) by Dr. Desgaultière. In this
gentleman I found a very enlightened physician,
who had had much experience, both in the army
and in private and hospital practice ; and, in the
present unsettled state of the opinions of medical
men about the cause of fever, his may be stated
here with propriety. I do this the more readily
as it appeared to me that his opinion was formed
not from any theoretical notions but from careful
and extensive observation, and because it ap-
proximates so closely to that which the great
increase of pathological researches has led so
many British practitioners of late to adopt. His
idea is that fever always depends upon local affec-

tion,—irritation or inflammation of some organ
or even an unusual accumulation of blood (con-
gestion) in some viscus without absolute inflammation.   He is far from limiting such local affection to the Gastro-Enteritic system with Dr.
Broussais ; yet his conviction is that fever invariably depends upon, and has its origin in some
local affection, and that from this we ought to set
out in our explanation of its phenomena.

   While on this subject I may mention a case,
stated to me by one of the physicians of the hospital, which shews the fallacy of some symptoms,
and the necessity of a very close attention to those
occurring in fever.   The case was that of a girl
attacked with acute fever accompanied with pain
in the epigastric region, so much increased by
pressure that she could scarcely suffer the region
of the stomach to be touched ;   there were also
symptoms of the brain being affected, but these
were considered rather as secondary and of less
consequence, the physician's principal efforts
being directed to relieve the supposed epigastric
affection.   The fever proved fatal, and, on examination, not the slightest mark of disease could
be detected in the stomach or bowels, which
were only slightly distended by air, but in the
brain the arachnoid membrane exhibited evident
marks of inflammation, and a considerable accu-

mulation of fluid had taken place in the ventri-
cles. Had this patient recovered, or not been
examined after death, no doubt would have existed on the mind of the medical attendant that
the stomach was the principal organ affected.

The other establishments of this kind in
Lyons are ' La Charité'—which is a receptacle
for Foundlings, a lying-in hospital for the un-
married, and a refuge for the aged and infirm
of both sexes,—and the ' Maison des Alienés.'
This latter building is well situated on the
southern declivity of mount Tourviers, and has
attached to it an hospital for Syphilitic and
Psora patients. The rooms for the deranged were pretty clean and well ventilated,
and the poor victims of this dreadful malady
are treated with lenity, and appeared pretty
comfortable. It contained sixty male, and a
hundred and fifty female patients ; and this,
I was told by the medical attendant, is nearly
in the usual proportion in which the sexes are
affected here. Among the female part he
informed me a great number of cases arose
from derangement of the uterine and lacteal
systems, and that of these more than two thirds
recovered—viz. about twenty four in thirty.
This establishment is about to be enlarged.

A A

In addition to these a public dispensary has been established in Lyons within the last twelve months, and there are also several ' Maisons de Santé' in the city, but none on a very respectable scale.

Such is the state of medical practice and the establishments for the cure or relief of disease in Lyons, as far as I was enabled to observe them during a residence of a few days. Incomplete as the account just given is, it must have been much more so, but for the attention and liberality of the medical officers of the different establishments, who afforded me every facility in my enquiries.

I was not a little surprized to find that in a military government, such as France has long been, there should be no military hospital at such a place as Lyons, but that the sick soldier should be obliged to seek refuge in the garrets of a civil hospital, already insufficient to supply the demands made upon it by the inhabitants.

It is also to be regretted that such an establishment as the Hotel Dieu, which has been endowed on a most liberal scale, should be burthened by a parcel of stout hale nuns and monks. A reasonable proportion of the former is a great acquisition to an hospital; as they are excellent nurses, and are very well in the

kitchen, conservatory, and such like ; but I
doubt much the propriety of their being allowed to have any thing to do with preparing
medicines : indeed one of the physicians remarked to me, while speaking of the practice,
that they were rather kept in check in prescribing
active medicines unless there was urgent necessity for it, for fear of mistakes, a proof of the
impropriety of such a custom, and a sad reflec-
tion upon the department of the Apothecary
of the Hotel Dieu. I shall conclude these remarks with two tabular views of cases treated
at this hospital during one year, from which
some idea of the number and also of the nature
of the diseases may be gathered ; though I am
sorry I am not able to give a more perfect report.

*Statement of patients received into the Hotel
Dieu of Lyons, in the six medical divisions,
between the* 1st *July* 1812, *and* 1st *July* 1813.

Men remaining in Hospital and received	
during the year	4,802
Women .... idem	5,093
Pregnant women .... idem	324
Total	10,219

Men discharged during same time or re-
maining July 1st, 1813 .... ,...... 4,281
Women .... idem   4,475
Women .... ' en couche' .... idem   317
Men deceased ....,....................... 521
Women .... idem ....,....................... 688
Women .... ' en couche' .... idem   7

Total 10,219

The following statement of patients treated
in Dr. Desgaultier's own division (one sixth of
the whole) will shew the proportion of the
various diseases during same period :

Fevers (1) 621	Organic Lesions (4) 495	
Phlegmasiæ (2) 527	Exanthemata	108
Homorrhagiæ (3) 43	Neuroses	189

Total 1983

(1) These are divided according to the system
of Pinel which Dr. D. would not do now.

(2) Including dysentery (of which there are
twenty five cases) and Catarrh.

(3) Including sanguine apoplexy.

(4) Under this division I have included
seventy three cases most of which were trifling
and of which thirty one were entitled ' Fatigues
de Route.'

The cases of consumption amount to one
hundred and nineteen and stand thus : —

Pulmonary consumption in men ... 80.
.... women ... 21.
————111
Laryngeal consumption in men .... 4.
.... women ... 3.
——— 7
Mesenteric consumption (all in males)   11
—————
Total 119

STRASBOURG.

Strasbourg forms one of the three medical schools of France, and a few years ago the number of medical students amounted to from four to five hundred. At present there are only about two hundred, and from thirty to forty only take their degrees annually.

At my visit there were only a few summer lectures going on, and the classes were very thinly attended. Dr. Foderé, professor of medical jurisprudence, &c. I found lecturing on the diseases of grain, and its effects on man, which had been of late severely felt at Strasbourg and its vicinity. Specimens of the diseased grain were handed round to the students. After the lecture I was accompanied by this learned physician to the Museum which is large and rich in pathological preparations. A catalogue is about to be published of its contents by Dr. Lobstein, just appointed professor of pathology. The hospital of Strasbourg is attached to the poor house, and is badly planned, as are also the clinical wards attached to the lunatic asylum.

Professor Foderé has given a full account of the bad arrangements of the latter in his medicine legale.*

The medical school of Strasbourg has twelve professors' chairs, of which I shall subjoin a list.†

I regret that an accident prevented me from obtaining the information and deriving the full advantages I expected from my short visit to this city. I cannot however conclude these very imperfect notes on Strasbourg without testifying my admiration of the very extensive acquirements of Professor Foderé, which indeed are already well known to the medical world through the medium

---

* When at Paris Dr. Esquirol informed me that a new lunatic asylum was about to be erected at Strasbourg, on the very excellent plan detailed in that gentleman's interesting report on the state of madhouses in France.

---

† *Lauth* .... Anatomy.
  Berot .... Physiology and Clinical Surgery.
  Caillot .... Pathology and Surgery.
  Cose .... Clinical Medicine.
  Flamand .... Midwifry and diseases of women and children.
  Foderé .... Medical jurisprudence and police, and epi-
                 demic diseases.
  Gerboin .... Materia Medica, and Theraputics.
  Lobstein .... Pathological Anatomy.
  Meunier .... Medical Hygiene.
  Masuyer .... Chemistry.
  Nestlet .... Botany, and Pharmacy.
  Jourdes .... Medical Pathology.

of his valuable publications,* though his affability
of manners and readiness in communicating his
knowledge may not be so well known   For his
kindness and attention to a perfect stranger I owe
him my grateful thanks. The reader will not think
the worse of Professor F., I presume. from knowing that he is a great admirer of English medicine.   He expresses his detestation of the system
of charlatanism carried on in a certain great continental capital, and laments much the little encouragement given to scientific pursuits in his
part of the country. As a proof of this I may
mention that he has had lying by him in a finished
state the very valuable work on the Maritime
Alps already noticed in the first part of this
essay. That country is, however, now little
interesting to France, and the new Government,
to which the work ought to be most interesting,
would probably not suffer it to be published in
its territory.†

* Professor Foderé is preparing for the press, a work on nervous
diseases, as a sequel to his work De Delire, and has in considerable for-
wardness another which is to form a supplement to his large work, and
a manual of medicine legale for the practitioner.

‡ A Piedmontese Gentleman of my acquaintance who had formed a
Geological map of the environs of Nice, with considerable labour, told
me he could not now venture to publish it, lest he should subject him.
self to the suspicion of the present Government.   To have been appointed a Professor in any of the Universities in that Country during
the late order of things, is now considered a sufficient crime to render
the individual incapable of holding his chair.

BOLOGNA.

The Medical School of Bologna ranks among the first of those in Italy. In some respects it is ill calculated for attracting a numerous concourse of Students, being placed almost at one extremity of the Papal States, and bordering on those of Austria, the youth of which latter are obliged to study at their own Universities.

Medicine at Bologna is cultivated with assiduity, and the Professors are men of established reputation. Tommasini, Professor of Medicine, is well known as the Author of an excellent work on Yellow Fever, and several others of less note. He is one of the great supporters of the new Italian, or *Contra-sti-mulant* doctrine, as it is called, and which, in practice at least, is directly opposed to the system of Brown, which for a long time was advocated warmly in Italy. The latter, it is well known, considered almost all diseases as arising from debility, and requiring Stimulants, while the present doctrine, ' Nuova Dottrina Medica Italiana' looks upon most diseases as arising from increased action, and requiring

B B

depriments—contra-stimulants. The medical
school of Bologna may be considered at the
head of this new doctrine, and the Professors
its most able and zealous advocates.*

The University is a handsome building.
The Museum of Natural History is extensive;
and there is, also, an Anatomical Museum,
chiefly of wax-work, similar, though much inferior to that of Florence. The collection of
obstetrical preparations in wax is large, and
was chiefly prepared by a female. The library
is large, and is open to the public every day,
from nine in the morning till two in the after-
noon ; as is the case in all the libraries of this
kind that I have met with on the continent.
Every convenience is afforded for reading books,
making extracts, &c. in the library, but none
are permitted to be taken out of it.

While noticing the library of Bologna, I
cannot avoid paying my tribute of respect to
the talents and acquirements of its librarian,
Professor Mezzofanti, one of the greatest lin-
guists now living.   Since the death of the late

* For an account of this system, I must refer the reader to the
small work of Tommasini " Della nuova Dottrina Medica Italiana."
A Periodical Journal is also just established at Bologua, for the express purpose of giving an account of the rise and progress of this
doctrine, entitled " Giornale Della nuova Dottrina, &c."

lady Professor of Greek, who died in 1816, he holds two chairs in this University, those of Greek and Oriental languages. He has already acquired a sufficient knowledge of thirty different languages, to enable him to converse in them, and is, besides, acquainted with several others. Among these may be mentioned the whole of those of Europe, several of the East, and those of Peru, Brazil, and Mexico. The general knowledge of this extraordinary man, appears to be very extensive.—Of the present state of the arts and sciences in England he is well informed ; and in speaking to him of the state of medicine, before he had introduced me to the medical professors, I found him perfectly acquainted with the present medical theories of Italy. He is allowed, annually, a small sum by the Government, for the purchase of books for the library, and a considerable proportion of this is laid out in English books of science. Professor Mezzofanti has been the means of establishing a taste for acquiring languages among the Bolognese, and I was informed that not a few young ladies were then learning English. He appears to be about forty years of age, and it is to be feared that his great assiduity in the discharge of his various duties will soon injure a constitution not naturally very strong. I hope I shall be excused these few words concerning this extraordinary and excellent man, whom all who have the pleasure of knowing cannot fail to admire and esteem.

There are altogether about two hundred medical students at the University of Bologna; but of these a small proportion only aspire to the higher ranks of the profession. Many, I found, were merely preparing themselves for being Apothecaries, and many to practise the lower branches of surgery—' Bassa Chirurgia,' —a class in the profession unknown among us, and holding a rank something similar to the ' officiers de santé,' in France.

This system of sending forth a set of half-educated men, who, no doubt, as in other countries, overstep in their practice, the limits prescribed to them, is, with justice, complained of by the regularly educated members of the profession in Italy: The Germans are blamed for introducing this practice. A system more calculated, indeed, to bring the profession into disrepute, cannot well be imagined; and it may be one, among several other causes, of the very different rank in society which the medical men of Italy hold, compared with those in England. But a still stronger reason may be found, I apprehend, in the system of gratuitous medical education in use in the former country. The students attend the lectures and hospitals almost for nothing, and the graduation fees are very trifling. The annual salary of the medical professors themselves, amounts only to about £150. The facility thus afforded to medical students of acquiring their profession on easier terms than the lowest mechanic can his trade, so common on the continent, and of which they boast, though it may have some advantages, is, upon the whole, I am inclined to believe, injurious to the profession.

The medical faculty consists of twelve chairs, the nature of which, with the names of their present occupiers are given in the Appendix.

The following is the plan of medical study prescribed by the laws of the University:

In Medicine.

First Year.—Natural History, Botany, General Chemistry, Anatomy.

Second Year.—Anatomy, Physiology, Comparative Anatomy, Institutes of Surgery.

THIRD YEAR.—Pathology, Clinical Medicine (as Spectators), Materia Medica, Pharmaceutical Chemistry.

FOURTH YEAR.—Pathology, Clinical Medicine (as Practitioners), Medical Jurisprudence, Midwifery, Veterinary Surgery.

In Surgery.

FIRST YEAR.—The same as in Medicine, with the addition of Pharmaceutical Chemistry.

SECOND YEAR.—Same as in Medicine.

THIRD YEAR.—Institutes of Surgery, Clinical Surgery (as Spectators), Materia Medica, Dissections and Operative Surgery.

FOURTH YEAR.—Clinical Surgery (as Operators), Dissections and Operative Surgery on the dead body, legal Medicine, Midwifery, Veterinary Surgery.

Both classes of students, during the last two years, are obliged to attend the hospital daily. At the termination of the first year, they take the degree of *Bachelor*, at the end of the second, that of *Licentiate*; at the termination of the course that of *Doctor* in Medicine or Surgery. Graduates of either class wishing to take the highest degrees in the other, must study an additional year.

The course of study prescribed for Apothecaries, and Veterinary Surgeons, is only for a couple of years. The following are the classes they must attend :

Apothecaries.

FIRST YEAR.—Natural History, Botany, General and Pharmaceutical Chemistry.

SECOND YEAR.—The same, and Materia Medica.

Veterinary Surgeons.

FIRST YEAR.— General and Pharmaceutical Chemistry, Comparative Anatomy, Elements of Veterinary Surgery.

SECOND YEAR.—Botany, Physiology, Veterinary Surgery.

These two classes of students, after the first year, take the degree of bachelor, and after the second, that of licentiate.

The mode of examination of candidates for the different degrees seems very judicious, and is considerably different from that followed in our medical schools. Five professors constitute a quorum, and at the examination of a can-

didate each submits to him twenty different
subjects taken from his own particular course of
instruction.   He draws one of these by lot, and
is forthwith examined upon it, whatever it may
be.   At the termination of the examination the
professors give their votes secretly,   and the
number of these obtained, and the mode in
which they are obtained, by the candidates,
constitute three different modifications of the
same   degree   which   are   expressed   in   the
diplomas.

If they obtain two thirds of the votes they
are declared *approved*; if the whole, they are
declared *unanimously approved* (a pieni voti);
and to express a still further praise they are
declared *honourably approved*—(approvati con
lodi): Those who are rejected cannot present
themselves till after another year's study.

I was told that the plan of study just described is about to be changed by an order from
Rome.

The Botanic garden is small, but kept in
excellent order by Professor Bertoloni, who is
the Author of several esteemed Works on
Botany.   There is also a small garden for agricultural experiments.

The general hospital is kept in good order,

but its situation is not unexceptionable, and I
was told sores often put on a bad appearance
and were difficult to heal in it. In my visits to
this hospital with the physician Dr. Medici,
professor of physiology, (to whom I am indebted
for many marks of attention,) 1 was rather surprized to find so very large a proportion of the
patients labouring under inflammatory affections
of the chest. They were mostly chronic.

Their treatment of pneumonia differs chiefly
from ours in taking away smaller quantities of
blood at a time, which necessarily requires the
evacuation to be more frequently repeated. This
does not appear to arise from a fear of taking away
too much blood, for they seem liberal enough in
the use of the lancet.* In all inflammatory affections the general febrifuge medicine is a solution of
tartrite of antimony, which they give in considerable doses. On enquiring its effects Dr. M.

---

* This practice is not peculiar to Bologna. On going round one
of the hospitals of Rome, with the physician, we came to a young ple-
thoric man labouring under inflammation of the lungs. He had been in
the hospital twenty-four hours and had been bled three times, twice to
seven, and once to six ounces, and had had four blisters applied, one
to each arm, and one to each thigh. On enquiring what he expected
from the numerous blisters, he said, they were contra-stimulants. It
appears to me that had the whole blood taken away at three times, been
taken at once, and the blisters omitted, this patient would have probably required little else. He came in on the attack of the disease.

C C

told me, that, though it occasionally acted in increasing some of the secretions, it was not given with that intention, but as a medicine, that, without any evident effect, diminished febrile action. I found both this physician and professor Tommasini particularly careful in examining the appearance and consistence of the crassamentum of the blood taken from their patients. It was turned from the vessel in which it was contained into another, and with the edge of the former cut through in several directions.

There were a few intermittent but no continued fevers in the hospital when I was there. The former I was told, had become more frequent since the culture of rice had been introduced into the country around Bologna, about twenty years ago. The culture of this grain requires the ground to be kept mostly under water, and thus gives rise to the production of the infectious miasmata, by creating an artificial marsh.

The clinical hospital is near the university, and I found it in very good order. It contains twenty four medical patients. These are selected from the general hospital, or received from the town. As the session was at a close there were only a few chronic cases remaining at the time of my visit, and these of little interest.

The contra-stimulant doctrine which is in so
high favour at Bologna, prevails, I believe,
more or less over the whole north of Italy. The
Brunonian theory, however, has still a few supporters, and I was told that the expectant system
prevailed at one University, not many years ago,
of much reputation. The clinical professor had
lately however begun to see that the physician
had something more to perform than the duty of
a nurse, in the treatment of acute diseases.

PADUA.

The University of Padua at present holds a deservedly high character in Italy, as a medical school.—Within the last few years, the number of students has considerably increased, and, the present building being found too small, the Emperor, on his late visit to Italy, gave orders for the erection of a new one, on a more extensive scale.   The plan of medical studies in the University of Padua is good.   It extends to five years ; and two courses of lectures are delivered in each Session.

The following is the plan of study :

In Medicine.

First Year.—Human Anatomy, and Elements of Medicine, and Surgery (in Latin), Natural History, Botany.

Second Year.—Anatomy, and Physiology (in Latin), General Animal and Pharmaceutical Chemistry.

Third Year.—General Therapeutics and

Materia Medica (in Latin), General Pathology,
Elements of Surgery, Midwifery.

FOURTH YEAR.—Clinical Medicine, Spe-
cial Therapeutics (in Latin), Veterinary Surgery.

FIFTH YEAR.—Continuation of two first
courses of last year, Medical Jurisprudence,
Medical Police, Diseases of the Eye, &c.

Surgery.

The course of instruction for Students in
Surgery is the same as the above for the first
three years.

FOURTH YEAR.—Practical Surgery, Veterinary ditto.

FIFTH YEAR.—Practical Surgery, Medical
Jurisprudence, Diseases of the Eye, Medical
Police.

Provincial Surgeons.

FIRST YEAR.—Anatomy, Physiology, Pathology, General Therapeutics, Materia Medica, and the writing of receipts.

SECOND YEAR.—Clinical Surgery, Internal
Diseases, Operative Surgery, Medical Jurisprudence, Midwifery, Veterinary Surgery.

Apothecaries.

One Year —Chemistry, Natural History, Botany.

Veterinary Surgeons.

First & Second Years.—Physiology, Pathology, and General Therapeutics, Theory of Agriculture, Theoretical and Practical Veterinary Surgery, Materia Medica, and writing of receipts.

Dr. Brera, the Professor of Medicine, is too well known for any thing I could say, to add to his high medical character, but I may be allowed to bear testimony to his no less frank and affable manners, and to acknowledge my obligations to him for several marks of personal attention.*

The general hospital of Padua, is a very excellent building, and the wards are commo-

---

* Professor Brera is at present engaged in a work on contagious diseases (*De' contagi e della cura de' loro effetti Lezioni medico-prattche*) He is also about to publish a new edition of Burserius's *Institutiones Medico Pratica* with notes, and also of his own excellent work on Intestinal worms.

dious, and kept in good order. This remark is particularly applicable to the Clinical wards, under the care of Professor Brera.*

Unfortunately from the session being almost finished, this department of the hospital contained only a few chronic cases   At his visit Dr. B. entered into a short history of, and made some remarks upon, each case.   In his remarks upon a case where Epistaxis and Hæmorrhois alternated with each other, on which occasion he made some very excellent observations on the affections of the vascular system, he related the case of a man so subject to vertigo, that to relieve himself he had recourse to bleeding every week . he was recommended to postpone the bleeding, but could never do so beyond the tenth day, without his feelings becoming intolerable to him.   He died of apoplexy.

In a case of a very painful affection of the hip joint, in which the bones were enlarged, and which had been treated for many years as

* The circumstance noticed in a former part of this work, when speaking of the Climate of Rome, namely, of the patients in the clinical wards being occasionally attacked by intermittent fevers, when the windows are incautiously left open at night, shews the situation of this hospital to be by no means unexceptionable.

rheumatism, the actual cautery had been applied upon Rust's plan, and by one application has relieved the pain; a cure I believe was not anticipated.

In two cases of cancer uteri, Professor B. was using the *extractum Calendulæ officinalis* * with an alleviation, at least, of the symptoms. This medicine, as well as the *extractum Cerefoliæ* he has frequently found useful in mitigating the painful symptoms of this dreadful disease, where opium had proved useless. He also employs a weak solution of the *aqua cohobatæ Laurocerasi* as an injection.†

It has been doubted by some, whether the plan of delivering clinical lectures at the bed-side of the patient, or in the lecture-room, is best suited for the improvement of the student. Both, no doubt, have their peculiar advantages, though the latter, upon the whole, appears to deserve the preference. The former, however, might still be adopted with advantage, so far as to call the particular attention of the student, to the cases or symptoms most worthy of remark,

* The calendula was found useful in cancer by Westrin.

† Vide " De Præcipuis Acidi Prussici et aquæ cohobatæ Laurocerasi medicis Facultatibus clinicis observationibus comprobatis Specimen. J. A. Manzoni Patavii 1818."

while the patient was under his immediate observation.

An excellent bath for the application of the fumes of sulphur had lately been erected in the hospital, and its employment had been found useful in several cases of cutaneous disease. I was aware before my visit to Padua that, by the warmer supporters of the New Italian doctrine, Professor Brera was considered but a luke-warm advocate of that system. I found, however, that upon the whole he thought well of it, but could not adopt it in its full extent; observing justly, that no system that had ever yet been invented was sufficient to guide the physician in a large proportion of the cases that come under his observation.

The botanic garden at Padua is very good, but like all those I have seen in Italy, deficient in variety of shade and exposure. As at Bologna, there is a piece of ground appropriated to agricultural experiments.

PAVIA.

Though my visit to this place was so short that I ought scarcely to mention it, still I cannot pass it by, were it only to pay my tribute of respect to the justly celebrated Scarpa. Every thing about the medical school of Pavia is very perfect, and the musea, class-rooms, &c. all arranged and fitted up in a very superior style; yet I was surprized to find every thing on so small a scale at a University, which, at one time collected so great a concourse of students from all parts of Europe and boasted of some of the first medical professors in the world.

As a medical school Pavia is now much fallen in estimation. The number of medical students of all classes in the session of 1817 and 1818, I was told, amounted to nearly four hundred, and that about forty annually took the higher degree of the profession. The wards of the general and clinical hospital were in good order, but small. We must not, however, forget that the town is but small, containing only about 20,000 inhabitants. This is a circumstance which must always have been against Pavia as a school of practical surgery. It ought, however, to add not a little to the merit of the venerable Scarpa, whose works have added so largely to the stock of surgical knowledge, and to whom this University is so much indebted.

Scarpa is now the director of the medical department of the University ; the plan of medical study at which, 1 shall not mention, as he informed me they are about to change it. Scarpa's sight has failed him much, yet he appears to enjoy good health, and a flow of spirits and cheerfulness not often met with at his age. Although in a great measure retired from the exercise of his profession, he has lost nothing of his enthusiasm for it. In his library, I found all the best English medical works. He complained much of the very tedious manner in which he received publications from our country, being obliged frequently to get them round by Germany It is much to be regretted that in the time of general peace which now exists, and which for the sake of science, had we no other motive, it is to be hoped may long exist, some means should not be adopted to facilitate communication in the literary world.

Whoever visits this great man will, in addition to the pleasure and information derived from his animated conversation, find in his house a collection of some of the finest paintings by the first Italian masters; for Scarpa is an admirer, and an encourager of the fine, as well as the useful, arts.

I cannot finish this subject without remarking that the whole that I have seen, conspires to impress me with the very superior state of activity with which medical science, and I might add, all the other sciences, is cultivated in the north of Italy, compared to what they are in the more southern parts. Of the state of medical practice beyond the Appenines I have said nothing, for several reasons, the principal of which is that I shall soon have more extensive opportunities of observation on that subject, and another occassion may offer of my making a few remarks on it.*

---

* Of the state of medical practice in the most celebrated of the places just alluded to, perhaps the following reply of the learned lady of a still more learned Baronet, may not convey a very incorrect idea: speaking of the * * * * * Doctors, a gentleman observed—that they dispatch their patients here *secundum artem* as well as elsewhere; —" No " returned her ladyship, " they kill here *secundum naturam.*"

TURIN.

HOSPITAL OF ST. JOHN.

This is the only general hospital of Turin.
It is a very handsome building, but, like many
other continental hospitals, is constructed on a
plan more calculated to produce an imposing
effect, than to satisfy the medical visitor. The
wards are distributed on the ground floor and
first story, the former being appropriated to the
men, the latter to the women. The form in
which they are disposed is that of a cross with
the addition of a large ward at the extremities
of two of the arms of the cross, the whole communicating so freely as almost to form but one
ward. These wards are large, lofty, and tolerably well lighted; but, owing to the windows
being very high, and no other means adopted
for ensuring a free circulation of air, they are
not very well ventilated. The floors are of
brick, which it is difficult even to make appear
clean. The only mode of warming the hospital
in winter is by means of large *choffers* containing live charcoal placed at certain distances,—
a plan not much calculated for improving the

state of the air. The beds are by no means
crowded; indeed, without being so, a much
greater number might have been admitted,
without having recourse to the central row,
which in these large wards is always done when
they are crowded with patients. The whole
number of patients in the hospital at my visit
(in October) amounted to four hundred and
eighteen,—the number of male and female
patients being nearly equal. The proportion of
surgical cases was small, there being only
seventy in all. In the number of patients,
however, are included a class of individuals
called Pensioners, (Pensionarii) who pay a
small sum for remaining in the hospital. They
amounted to nearly one third of the whole, and
the greater number was, apparently, without
any complaint, or at least disease. The cases
in the hospital consisted chiefly of a chronic
nature, with a few slight continued, and a few
intermitted fevers. Epidemics are very rare
at Turin; The most prevalent diseases are of
the inflammatory kind. Phthisis Pulmonalis
without being particularly frequent is by no
means an unfrequent disease. The medical establishment of St. John's consists of four ordinary
physicians, and two assistant physicians, (who remain at the hospital to examine and receive pa-

tients;) two surgeons and six surgical elèves.
During the session, the clinical professors have
also their patients in this hospital, ten being
allowed to each. The funds of this hospital, I
was told were good. It is governed by the
clergy who regulate the admission of the Pensionarii.

The following report of the state of St.
John's for 1818 is the only kind of one that
could be obtained or was made.

Report of St. John's Hospital, Turin, for 1818.

	Men.	Women.	Total
Remaining 31st Dec. 1817	219....	261....	480
Received during the year	2,359....	1,721....	4,080
Total	2,578....	1,982....	4,560
Discharged during the year	2,072....	1,531....	3,603
Died	289....	199 ...	488
Total	2361....	1,730....	4,091
Remaining 31st Dec. 1818	217....	252....	469

LA CARITA.

This is an Establishment applied to various uses; it forms at once a refuge for those unfortunate children deserted by their parents, from poverty or other causes, who are sent here directly from the town, or from the foundling hospital as soon as they can work; for those afflicted with epilepsy, and other incurable diseases; and it also forms an hospital for the syphilitic and psora patients who are not admitted into the general hospital. This, it must be confessed, is a singular enough admixture of subjects. The building consists of two large courts united together, one for males, and another for females. The whole number in this immense establishment amounted to two thousand five hundred. The greater number were young, and they were all employed at work, chiefly cotton and woollen manufatures, and upon the whole, appeared in good spirits and healthy looking. I went over the whole establishment, and I must say it is far from being in the state it ought to be. The upper parts are occupied for sleeping chambers, the ground floor for work rooms. The air in these last was generally in a very impure state, little attention being paid to regular ventilation. Altogether, I fear, the intentions which the founders of this Institution had on its formation, are not so well fulfilled as they might be.

CASA DE' PAZZI—LUNATIC ASYLUM.

My expectations of this Establishment were
not raised very high, from the state in which I
found that which I have just mentioned, and still
less from some conversation I had with one of
the medical professors of the university the evening preceding my visit, (during which I perceived
evidently a wish that I should not see it,) but
I never could have anticipated the dreadful spectacle of tortured humanity which was here exhibited, and of which any description I can give
must come far short of the impression it made
upon my mind. I shall simply state the situation
of the wards and patients as I found them at the
time of my visit.

The part of the hospital we were first taken
to consisted of small rooms, similar to those generally met with in such institutions, but I was
disappointed to find these were not for the
poor patients, but for those who paid a certain
sum for being kept. The first of these that was
opened presented to us the wretched prisoner perfectly naked, and chained down to his bed by
both wrists. He had raised himself up in his bed
as far as his chains admitted, by which movement
he had thrown off the single coverlet that had been
cast over him. He had no shirt; his legs (ap-

parently red and swollen from cold) were drawn
up under the corner of the bed-cover, which lay
over a small part of his body ; he was pale and
emaciated ; he uttered not a word. In short a
human being in so wretched a state I had never
before seen ; but I was soon to witness others in
a state still more horrible.

We were next conducted into a ward where
thirty beds were huddled together, on most of
which lay a poor wretch chained by one or more
limbs to the bedstead ; for to each corner of these
was attached a massy iron chain, with a clasp of
the same materials and strength at the extremity,
for admitting the wrists and ankle; and, according as the keeper judged necessary, one or more
of these were applied. Some were polished and
bright as silver, from constant use. I imagined
these were their most unruly patients, but was
told that this was by no means the case.

To these we were next led; and on the un-
bolting of the door of a large cell, the scene that
presented itself almost exceeds belief. The spectacle of the poor wretches, naked, or covered only
by some straw, chained down hand and foot to
their bedsteads,—the clanking of their chains,—
the dreadful vociferations they set up at the sight
of him who rivetted these chains,—and still more,
the horror excited by such a spectacle, no terms

are strong enough to depict! I had read and
heard of chains and other means of torture for
subduing (irritating,) the unfortunate Maniac; I
had even seen such singly chained to the wall
by the neck like an infuriated and dangerous
beast;—but a den like this, crowded and
crammed with human beings, chained down,
without a rag of covering, struggling to raise
their heads and exhibiting their emaciated and
galled limbs from the heap of straw that had
been thrown upon them, was a scene I never
expected to witness, and which I hope in God
I may never witness again! After visiting similar establishments in Paris, and some in our own
country, where chains have been laid aside, and
a mild system of treatment adopted, with a success which (setting humanity out of the question) more than warrants its continuance, I was
ill prepared to meet such a dreadful contrast on
crossing the Alps. In this cell there were
twelve men, three of whom only were allowed
any thing more than straw to cover them.
Some I was told had been confined there for
many months. On approaching them they exhibited their chained limbs with the most earnest
entreaties for liberation. One man had two
chains on one arm. In this case the space
between the iron clasps was red, swollen, and

ulcerated, and the mortification, which in all
probability was to follow, would soon render
chains unnecessary for him. Others had their
limbs galled, but not in such a degree as that
described. In one instance only in the whole
hospital did I observe any thing introduced
between the iron ring and the limb. The rest
of the men's wards were similar to that I first
noticed.

From the men's we were led into the
women's department, which was in the higher
part of the house, and which, in every respect,
we found similar to that we had just left,—the
beds huddled closely together, chains—always
ready—many applied, and most of the beds
occupied ; for whether to save trouble, or from
the poor creatures having no clothes but the
coverlet that was thrown over them, almost
every one was in bed. Here, as below, was also
a cell where straw afforded the only covering,
where the chains were more heavily applied, and
where the state of furious desperation to which
the wretched victims were driven, was expressed
in terms equally violent and still more affecting.
One of these tortured women held up her arm
which was raw and had been bleeding, from
the iron clasp having worked its way into the
flesh !

Such is the dreadful state of this house, which contains one hundred and eighty males and ninety-seven females, of whom one third the keeper told me, were kept *constantly* chained. From the same source I learned that the annual number of deaths (and this I apprehend is the principal way in which this house gets rid of its inhabitants;) sometimes amounted to eighty, (nearly one third of the whole); that they *had* been as few as thirty; and that the average was fifty, (nearly one fifth)—a mortality I believe unequalled in any institution of the kind in any country. The only good thing I observed about this establishment was a piece of ground which had just been enclosed for the exercise of those whose chains were permitted to be undone.

Such is the state of the institutions at Turin for the refuge and relief of afflicted humanity. St. John's, though by far the best regulated, and in the best order, affords ample room for improvement. The plan of admitting pensioners in a general hospital, is, I conceive, essentially a bad one, were it only as interfering with that regular system of order and uniformity which ought to be kept up in such an establishment. This hospital might also be cleaner and better ventilated. Of 'La Carita the plan is radically

bad. Syphilitic and cutaneous diseases should
never be admitted into such an establishment.
The house is generally dirty, in some places extremely so, and also badly ventilated, particularly
where the people were at work.—The very courts
which the building enclosed, and which should
be gravelled, and kept dry for the exercise of the
young in the intervals of their working hours,
were overgrown with weeds, or covered with
filth and rubbish, and, from their extreme humidity, more calculated to produce than prevent
disease.

With respect to the murderous receptacle for
the deranged, I know not what relief to propose;
nothing but a perfect change, I fear, can remedy
the state it is in; perhaps it would even be for
the benefit of humanity, that the same dreadful
remedy were applied to it as was formerly applied
to the Hotel Dieu of Paris; and could it rise
from its ashes in *Piedmont* as that hospital did
in France, he who applied the torch would
deserve to be ranked among the benefactors of
his country and mankind. In its present state,
it is an infamous disgrace to the Government
under which it exists :—I say Government,
because, in a despotic one, such as that of
Piedmont, where private opinion dares not be
expressed, the Government alone is responsible

for the state of all such institutions. But these things are beneath the notice of a King of Sardinia (who, by the way, is particularly bound to visit La Carita in person; but he prefers a deputy, who again, I fear, employs a substitute, in imitation of his magnanimous Sovereign). The royal family of France are not ashamed, in their visits to the departments, to look into the Hospitals, and even to administer consolation at the bed-side of their sick subjects; Napoleon and his ministers did the same; and the Emperor of Austria, in his late journeys, visited the hospitals as well as other public institutions: but such is the horror of an hospital at the court of Sardinia, that a physician who has entered one, is not suffered to cross the precincts of the palace, lest he should carry the seeds of infection among the royal family !

GENOA.

The general hospital of Genoa partakes of the grandeur of the other buildings of that once wealthy city. Its magnificent marble stair-cases,—the large court round which it is built, with its arcades supported on beautiful marble pillars, produce a very imposing effect, and 'at once evince the liberality and taste of its' benefactors, whose statues, also, ornament its walls.' The wards of this hospital are very large, but although tolerably well lighted, owing to the height at which the windows are placed, (which without the employment of other means renders the circulation of air difficult,) it is not very well ventilated. The width of the wards is such, that there were occasionally in them three, and sometimes four ranges of beds, (placed lengthwise across the ward) without being very much crowded.

All diseases are admitted into this hospital. There are two wards for children, and a part of the house is set apart as a lying-in-hospital. The small-pox ward contains only two cases. Cow-pox inoculation is much neglected here, but I was told it had just begun to be more at-

tended to. The floors of this hospital are of
brick and were not particularly clean ;—the
bedsteads are of iron and no curtains are used.
Baths are attached to the hospital.† The number of patients at the time of my visit (in October) to this hospital, was four hundred and forty
females, and three hundred and sixty males;—of
these one hundred and twenty-eight were surgical cases. The medical establishment consists of four ordinary physicians and four as-

* During the time of the French, vaccination was particularly
well attended to in all this country. Since they left it it has been neglected like too many other things, and it was only in August last that
the present Government took any steps to spread the benefits of vac
cination among its subjects.

† The manner of preserving their leeches at this hospital may be
mentioned. They are kept in a large stone trough or basin, at the
bottom of which there is some sand and gravel, and in which the
water is constantly renewed by a very small stream entering it
through a tube, and a similar quantity being allowed to escape,—the
whole completely exposed to the air. In this way they find the leeches
not only live but multiply abundantly, while in former practice, they
were constantly dying when kept in the bottles. The leeches which
are once used they invariably throw away, as they have found by experience that many of these not only died but injured the others when
returned. M. Major the chemist, I also found, kept his leeches in a
similar way. I have the more satisfaction in noticing any means for
the better preserving of these useful little animals, as what I have seen
on the continent certainly induces me to think more highly of the good
effects to be derived from the local abstraction of blood than most
English medical men are inclined to do at present.

sistant physicians, (one of whom is always at the hospital to receive patients,) four surgeons, and four assistants.

The most prevalent diseases of Genoa are inflammatory affections of the chest—pulmonary consumption being a very frequent disease. This they attribute to the very variable nature of their climate. Examinations after death in particular cases only are put in practice here. There is a theatre in the hospital for anatomical demonstrations. The medical practice, judging from what I was told and observed, differs little from the system adopted in the French hospitals.

SPEDALE DEGLI INCURABILI.

The other Hospital of Genoa is appropriated to incurable chronic diseases—epilepsy, mania, &c. and upon the whole appeared fully in as good a state as the general hospital. The whole number of patients in this hospital amounted to seven hundred, of which four hundred and fifty were females, and two hundred and fifty males. The more prevalent diseases were chronic catarrhal affections and chronic rheumatism.— There was one ward filled by boys, and another by girls, who were scrophulous, almost without an exception; and yet scrophula, I was informed, except as affecting the lungs, is not considered a very frequent disease at Genoa. Cancer is also rare; in the whole of this hospital I was informed, on enquiry, there were only six cases of that disease.

The difference in this respect, and also in the progress of pulmonary consumption, between Marseilles and Genoa is worthy of remark: both places lie in the same latitude, both stand on the shores of the Mediterranean, and the productions of both are very similar. The climate of Genoa, (though I have not yet had sufficient opportunity of comparing them) is somewhat more moist than that of Marseilles, yet both are dry;

intermittents being almost unknown in either.
Now, at Genoa, cancer is a rare disease; at
Marseilles a very frequent and, of course, fatal,
as it very often attacks the uterus. In both
places consumption is very common; in Marseilles the progress of this disease is very rapid,
in Genoa very slow,—from three to four years,
I was informed, being its usual course.

The number of deranged in this hospital was
sixty women and fifty-five men. The women were
all kept in one large ward, with the exception
of a few who pay and have small rooms; these,
as well as forty epileptics in an adjoining ward,
were under the care of five nurses. The men
were in two adjoining wards. Chains I found
also in pretty frequent use in this institution,—
half the men (at my visit) and one third of the
women being chained. The chains however
were much less heavy than at Turin. All the
patients were also clothed here, and, upon the
whole, much more lenity seemed shewn to the
unfortunate patients than in the horrid establishment of that city. When so many of these
patients are kept together in one ward, either
some means of restraint seems necessary, or a
much larger number of attendants than is generally allowed. Other means of restraint, however, might be found besides chains.

Report of the General Hospital of Genoa for 1818 :

	Men.	Women.	Total.
Received during 1818	4155	4382	8537
Discharged, ditto ditto	3684	3977	7661
Died	531	636	1167

The population of Turin and Genoa is nearly the same, being about 80,000.—The number of patients admitted into the general hospital of the latter place is nearly twice as great as that of the former; but it must be stated that that of Genoa includes a lying-in-hospital and receives syphilitic and cutaneous diseases. The mortality is nearly the same in both—about one in seven and a half.

MEDICAL SCHOOLS OF TURIN AND GENOA.

The medical schools of these two places are placed together, because little need be said about either in their present state. Both are nearly in the same depressed condition, compared to what they were some time ago, and in both there are at present some prospects of improvement.

I believe it is not generally known, that, on the return of the present King of Sardinia, those Professors of Turin, and of his newly-acquired property, Genoa, who had been appointed to their chairs, during the time of the French Government, or whose talents had even been recognised and approved by it, were dismissed from these Universities. Twenty-five were displaced at Turin, and five at Genoa. How far the Government of his Sardinian Majesty was influenced by a love of science in this arbitrary act, may be seen from referring to a few of the names of those Professors, and from the state of those two Universities at present, compared with what they were in the time of the French Government. Among the former it will only be necessary to mention Balbis, the professor of botany at Turin, who now fills the chair of Decandolle at Montpellier; Jubert, who has lately been offered the chemical chair at Pavia, vacant by the death of Brugnatelli;—Gagliuffi, known as one of the most eminent Latin Scholars of Europe ; Multedo, who had filled the mathematical chair at Genoa with much reputation for twenty-four years, and whose talents induced Napoleon to call him to Paris, to assist in the arrangement of the weights and measures of that country; Dr. Mojon, Professor of Anatomy and Physiology at Genoa, who gained his chair by *concours* among twenty-four competitors as one of whom it is only necessary to mention, Tommasini, the present celebrated professor of medicine at Bologna.

How these professors have been replaced may be seen from the character which these schools now hold in Italy, and from the way they are attended.* The students at Genoa from upwards of four hundred, have now sunk to one hundred and fifty ; the medical students from eighty, to about thirty. We have only to compare, also, the Theses of the medical graduates during the time of the dismissed professors, and those at present produced, to perceive at once the different state of

---

* A medical practitioner in a village of Sardinia has a chair in one of these Universities, and from all the information I received, (and from a good source) he is as capable of filling any chair in the University as that which he now occupies.

these in the two periods. Formerly the candidates framed Essays upon particular subjects, like those of Edinburgh, several of which I have seen very creditable to their Authors and School: at present they are not Theses, but portions of the Professor's Lectures, one half of which is taken up from their dictation. This is the case at both Universities. At Turin, all the lectures are in Latin, a proof of itself how the profession is taught. No medical museum exists at either of these Universities at present. Not one anatomical preparation of any kind, I was told, is to be found at Turin. I must not omit to mention, however, while relating this sad lapse, the museum of Natural History at the Academia of Turin, which is a very respectable one, and in very excellent order. The cryptogamiæ have been admirably imitated here in wax, by an ingenious monk of Camaldoli, in the same way, and almost with equal truth, as the thick-leaved plants have been imitated at Florence. For such purposes, wax is admirably fitted, and its durability equals its other good qualities.*

---

* The application of wax to represent natural appearances is no where more useful or valuable than in the case of morbid anatomy. At Marseilles I have noticed its application to this purpose ; in the Museum of L'Ecole de Medecine at Paris, there are also some good representations of diseased structure preserved by this means ; but at

This museum is the only thing of the kind the scientific stranger will find to admire at Turin There is no literary, no medical periodical publications in his Sardinian Majesty's dominions, (if I except the memoirs of the academy of Turin, of which a volume is published annually,) and no medical Societies. Formerly, at Genoa, there was a highly respectable one, (Societá Medica di Emulazione) of which six volumes of memoirs were published, which were held in sufficient estimation to be translated into French.

In such a sad state of these Universities, it is some satisfaction to know that even the Government of Sardinia could not shut their eyes to it altogether, and those of the former professors who can be got, and who will accept of the office, are to be recalled forthwith. Some of these are determined not to accept of an apointment which they hold only by the caprice of the minister, unless they have some surety that they are not to be dismissed without trial.

---

no part in the Continent have I seen any thing to equal the wax preparations of morbid parts, by Mr. Charles Bell, in the excellent Museum in Great Windmill-Street, for the accuracy and fidelity with which the natural appearances are represented. It is only to be regretted that they are not more numerous.

APPENDIX.

No. 1. MARSEILLES. (Page 11.)

Principal Results of Observations made at the Imperial Observatory, Marseilles, for the Ten Years from 1796 to 1805 Inclusive. By M. Thulis.

		1796	1797	1798	1799	1800	1801	1802	1803	1804	1805	Mean of Ten Years.
Barometer, French inch and Lines	Highest	28 6 8	28 7 9	28 6 9	28 6 0	28 6 0	28 6 3	28 3 9	28 5 7	28 5 8	28 5 4	28 6 57 ·6
	Lowest	27 3 5	27 4 7	27 3 4	27 3 0	27 3 2	27 3 7	27 1 0	26 11 2	27 4 0	27 0 4	27 2 75
	Mean	28 1 30	28 1 20	28 1 42	28 0 44	28 0 60	28 0 12	28 0 30	27 8 40	28 0 00	27 8 9	27 11 95
Farenheit's Thermom.	Highest	84 425	91 625	84 65	83 3	93 2	86 45	99 275	99 375	99 275	90 125	90 77
	Lowest	26 15	22 775	31 775	17 6	17 375	29 075	23 85	21 65	23 85	30 425	25 45 27
	Mean	59 31	59 6075	59 135	53 535	60 4175	60 6575	60 55	58 55	59 2475	53 37	59 36
Quantity of Rain French inches & Lines		13 7	25 7	24 4 6	15 0 5	17 17	12 5 2	19 117	25 0 3	23 5 0	18 9 8	19 6 48 ·0
Prevailing Winds ..		N.W.W. S.W.	N.W. S.E.	N.W.E. S.E.	N.W. S.W.	N.W. S.E.	N.W.	N.W.	N.W.	N.W.	N.W.	N.W.
Rain		45	74	45	66	59	49	49	65	39	48	54
High Winds ..		52	43	29	31	29	29	22	156	102	99	57
Mist		11	3	15	13	5	10	1	1			6
Clear		94	59	107	74	73	66	109	108	91	105	92
Overcast		44	22	52	65	92	99	46	72	47	54	58
Cloudy		227	284	206	227	205	170	210	186	227	206	215
Frost		3	4	1	9	14	3	13	15	6		7
Snow		5	2	2	4	1	5	3	3	2		3
Hail			2	2	1	1			1			1
Thunder		7	14	25	9	9	8	7	7	6	4	10

Days

No. 2. MARSEILLES.

Mean Results of Three Years, (1807, 1808, 1809.) for the Winter Months (from October to March Inclusive) from Observations, by M. Thulis.

Month	Farenheit's Thermometer					Rain.	Snow.	Hail.	Fair.	Prevailing Winds.
	Mean.			Absolute.						
	Highest Degree.	Lowest Degree.	Mean Heat.	Max.	Min.					
Jan.	55 33	33 28	44 87	58 33	30 87	3 67	..	..	27 33	N. W.
Feb.	56 53	32 83	45 06	60 35	27 5	2 33	.33	..	25 33	N. W.
March	61 92	36 19	49 07	63 70	32	6	.33	..	24 67	N. W.
October	72 21	42 57	58 26	72 73	41	4	..	..	27	N. W.
Nov.	63 41	35 89	50 38	65 3	31 1	7 33	.67	..	22	N. W.
Dec.	56 14	28 33	46 56	57 87	23	4 67	.33	.33	25 67	N. W.
Mean	60 92	34 85	49 03			4 67	.28	.055	25 39	

APPENDIX.

No. 3. HIERES. (Page 23.)

State of the Weather at Hieres during the Months of February and March 1818, from the Observations of Mr. GAMBLE.

Feby 1818	Therm. Sunrise	Therm. Noon	Therm. Evening	Winds	REMARKS, &c.
1	43	56	44	West	Fine and Clear
2	45	53	41	Do.	Heavy Rain. P. M. Mistral
3	41	48	42	Do.	Thick & Cloudy. P. M. Rain
4	47	58	47	Do.	Clear Sunshine
5	50	58	47	N. W.	Clear and Fine
6	46	58	52	S. E.	Clear Strong Breeze
7	52	60	53	Do.	High Winds
8	52	59	53	Do.	Cloudy and Windy
9	54	61	54	Do.	Clear. P. M. a Gale
10	57	59	51	Do.	Bright Sunshine
11	48	61	51	Variable	Cloudy. P. M. Clear
12	47	59	45	N. W.	Do. Do.
13	45	50	41	E. N. E.	Stormy
14	41	38	42	Do.	High Wind [moderate
15	46	53	47	Do.	Cloudy, High Wind. P. M.
16	47	55	49	Do.	Fresh Breezes
17	48	59	49	Do.	Fine and Clear
18	45	61	47	Calm	Do. Do. Light Breeze
19	46	60	46	Variable	Do. P. M. Cloudy with Rain
20	46	59	52	Westerly	Constant Rain
21	54	56	50	S. W.	Cloudy, some rain, P. M. fine
22	50	59	52	N. W.	Very Strong Gale
23	50	52	46	Do.	High Winds [shine
24	46	59	49	Do.	Strong Breeze, Clear Sun-
25	40	63	51	Westerly	Fine
26	48	61	46	North	
27	44	52	47	Do.	
28	54	59	48		Windy with bright Sun

March 1818	Sunrise	Noon	Evening	Winds	REMARKS,
1	50	67	54	West	Bright Sunshine
2	51	63	49	Do.	Fine, some Clouds
3	50	60	54	East	Fine and Clear
4	54	61	52	S. W.	Rain, P. M. Fair
5	54	59	56	South	Cloudy
6	56	57	52	Do.	Hazy, with Rain
7	45	59	52	N. W.	Clear, P. M. fair & moderate
8	52	62	52	N. W.	Clear, High Wind
9	50	58	50	N. W.	Clear, P. M. Rain and Wind
10	51	61	55	West	Fine
11	48	55	48	North	Overcast, small Rain
12	50	59	53	West	Clear
13	49	59	46	N. W.	Clear
14	46	56	45	North	Clear
15	46	58	57	Vble	Small Rain
16	51	57	49	Do. P.M. NW.	Rain, P. M. Clear
17	49	61	51	North	Clear and Fine
18	55	68	55	Vble	Beautiful Clear Weather
19	48	65	51	North	Do. light airs
20	51	63	54	Vble	Do.
21	54	70	55	N. W.	Do.
22	54	63	52	Vble	Do.
23	52	64	52	Vble	Do.
24	52	63	55	South	Fine at times—Cloudy
25	53	59	50	N. W.	Fine
26	50	62	54	N. W.	Do. Windy
27	51	54	46	N. N. W.	Strong Mistral
28	46	61	46	N. E.	Fine and Clear
29	46	59	46	West	Do.
30	44	60	48	Do.	Do.
31	48	63	47	Do.	Do.

The material originally positioned here is too large for reproduction in this reissue. A PDF can be downloaded from the web address given on page iv of this book, by clicking on 'Resources Available'.

No. 4. NICE. (*Page* 36.)

Mean Results of Three Years, (1815—16—17—18) for the Six Winter Months, from the Observations of Mr. Risso.

Month.	Fahrenheit's Thermometer.						Rain	Snow	Hail	Fair	Prevailing Winds
	Mean.				Absolute.						
	Sunrise.	2. P. M.	Sunset.	Of 3 Preceding.	Max.	Min.					
Jan.	44 19	52 94	48 3	48 48	58 32	30 42	4	.67	..	26 33	N & NE
Feb.	47 62	57 49	52 14	52 42	63 28	40 77	1	..	..	27	NE. & SE.
March	50 81	61 09	55 14	55 88	66 42	43 25	2 23	..	..	28 67	NE.
Oct.	60 75	69 8	64 83	65 13	79 93	49 78	6	..	..	25	NE. & SE.
Nov.	51 35	62 43	56 06	56 61	70 02	39 43	4 33	..	..	25 67	N.
Dec.	44 06	56 16	48 77	49 66	63 73	36 5	3	..	.33	27 67	N & NE.
Mean	49 79	60 09	54 21	54 7			3 89	111	.055	26 72	

H H

No. 5. PISA. (Page 65.)

Mean Results of Three Years (1814—15—16,) for the Six Winter Months, from the Observations of Professor Zannini.

Month	Farenheit's Thermometer						Rain	Snow	Hail	Fair	Prevailing Winds
	Mean				Absolute.						
	Sunrise	2 P. M.	Sunset	Of 3 Preceding	Max.	Min.					
January	40 71	46 67	44 78	44 08	60 06	22 55	12	2	.03	16 7	N. E.
Feb.	43 41	51 26	48 74	47 79	58 55	20 75	11	·	·	17	N. E.
March	48 63	56 66	53 02	52 77	66 88	34 7	8	·	.06	22 4	N. E.
Oct.	60 82	66 11	62 78	63 23	77 ..	47 79	12	·	·	19	NE & NW
Nov.	49 95	55 4	53 62	52 99	66 43	35 15	18	0 3	·	11 7	N. E.
Dec.	42 94	48 29	46 51	45 91	57 65	22 77	16	·	.03	14 7	N. E.
Mean	47 74	54 06	51 57	51 13			12 83	0 34	.02	16 91	

No. 6. ROME. (Page 70.)

Mean Result of Three Years, (1815—16—17) for the Six Winter Months, from Observations by Professor Conti, of the Collegio Romano.

N. B. Thermometer is placed 70 feet above the Surface.

Month	Mean				Absolute		From	Rain	Snow	Hail	F air.	Prevailing Wind in Winter is the North.
	7. A. M	2, P. M	9. P. M	Of 3 Preceding.	Max.	Min.						
October	55 4	68 23	60 35	61 32	76 78	43 92	.	15	.	.	16	
Nov.	49 33	58 32	53 15	53 5	69 12	33 8	.	15	.	1	14	
Dec.	42 06	50 52	46 11	46 22	62 12	29 52	3	12	.	1	18	
Jan.	41 38	49 1	44 98	45 16	59 45	27 72	3	15	1	1	14	
Feb.	43 68	53 37	48 58	48 53	64 62	27 5	1	9	.	1	18	
March	47 75	57 71	51 06	52 18	66 65	35 15	.	9	.	1	21	
Mean	46 6	56 21	52 37		76 78	27 5					.	

The observation regarding the temperature of St. Peter's (stated P, 76) is not quite correct. The temperature of this church varies ten degrees throughout the year.

(No. 7. Page 52.)

Annual Returns of the Principal Diseases of the Mediterranean Fleet extracted from the Hospital Books.

MALTA.

DISEASE	No of Cases Received			No of Cases Invalided			No Died		
	1810	1811	1812	1810	1811	1812	1810	1811	1812
Phthisis Pulmonalis	56	58	35	13	28	16	34	21	12
Pneumonia	20	22	10	6	4	3	1	2	2
Fever	100	392	255	1	16	3	13	9	8
Flux		2							
Dysentery	13	14	9	4	4	2	4	2	3
GIBRALTAR									
Phthisis Pulmonalis	106	56	25	44	34	17	39	16	6
Pneumonia	10	23	18	3	4	6	1	4	3
Fever	71	23	44	2	8		10	3	4
Flux	16	2		2	1		6	1	
Dysentery	17	26	18	5	10	2	4	8	1
MINORCA									
Phthisis Pulmonalis		8	111			51		1	22
Pneumonia		5	32			10		2	5
Fever		53	304		3	10			11
Flux			9						4
Dysentery		37	14			2			

N. B. No Hospital Established at Minorca until the close of 1811.

(No. 8. Page 91.)

MEDICAL SCHOOL OF PAVIA.

PROFESSORS

Caldani .... Elements of Medicine—Human Anatomy (Latin)

Renier .... Natural History

Bonato .... Botany

Gallini .... Anatomy (higher) & Physiology

Melandri .... General, Animal, and Pharmaceutical Chemistry

Dalla-Decima ...... General Therapeutics, General Pathology, & Materia Medica

Dalle Ore .... Theory of Surgery

Ruggieri .... Midwifery, Clinical and Operative Surgery

Brera .... Clinical Medicine and Special Therapeutics

Molin .... Veterinary Surgery

Fanzago .... Medical Jurisprudence

Malacarne .... Physiology, Pathology, General Therapeutics, Materia Medica, Surgery and writing of receipts (for Provincial Surgeons)

Montesanto .... Internal Diseases (for Provincial Surgeons)

Arduino .... Agriculture (for Veterinary Surgeons)

Fabris .... Midwifery (for Midwives.)

(No. 9. Page 112.)

Extract of a Letter from Dr. Clark, dated Rome, December 25th, 1819, containing the following Extract of a Letter from Mr. Quadri to him, dated Naples, December 20th, 1819:

"*THE friend who interested himself in procuring me the opportunity of prosecuting my method of treating Goitre having left Naples, I have neglected, in some measure, this branch of practice; though I still cherish the hope of being able to reduce it to a certain degree of perfection. Reflecting on my past experience, I find that all Goitres of a soft consistence, and not arterial, were cured quickly and safely. (i. e. by the Seton). Of twelve individuals on whom the operation was performed, eight were perfectly cured. One patient being detained many weeks in the Hospital on account of the hard and indolent nature of the tumour, was attacked by Typhus Petechialis of which she died. Another very unmanageable patient with the swelling of the same indolent (freddo) and uninflammable nature, tore out the Seton; a fistula formed, accompanied by caries of the os hyoides and destruction of the organs of speech, which terminated in the death of the woman.*"

[These two cases, Mr. Quadri justly remarks, by no means militate against his method.]

"*The cases however must be distinguished in which this operation may be had recourse to with* *the greatest prospect of success; because in those cases where suppuration is excited with difficulty, and where much time is required, the patient is liable to the accidents which occurred in the two cases already stated.* In goitres of a hard firm structure the operation has been of little utility. In the Aneurismatic goitre, (Gozzo Aneurismatico) I should be inclined to practice the method of Walther, but in the soft goitre I should have no doubt about adopting my own. Thus far I can speak from the experience I have had, but I hope soon to have additional opportunities of observation on this subject.*"

From the above it appears that I have been misinformed, and that Mr Quadri still retains the same opinion of the utility of his practice, as when he sent the communication you mention to Dr. Somerville. We also learn from it that two circumstances in the nature in the goitre must be particularly attended to before adopting Mr. Quadri's plan—First that the tumour be of a soft texture, and sufficiently irritable to be thrown easily into the suppurative inflammation, and secondly that it be not of the Aneurismatic species.

J. C.

---

* The result of these two cases, and the circumstance of Mr. Quadri having ceased to continue his trials for some time, no doubt gave rise to the report (which was related to me as a fact) that he had abandoned the operation altogether. The result of the two remaining cases of the twelve, Mr. Quadri does not mention in his Letter

(No. 10.   Page 88.)

The physician alluded to p. 88. was my much respected colleague Dr. Slaney. I have no doubt that he
caught the fever by sleeping one night at Boccano on
his way from Rome to Florence in the end of July.
Boccano is a solitary post-house, situated in a low
swampy valley about twenty miles from Rome, noted
for its insalubrity. Dr. de Matthaeis, in the work
alluded to, calls it ' luogo d' aria la piu infame nelle
vicinanze di Roma'—of this Dr. S. was well aware
and was chiefly induced to risk sleeping in a place of
such danger from the fear of injuring an invalid (travelling with him) by proceeding during the night.

It has been said that Dr. S. fell a victim to the
disease, from his not believing in the malaria but I
know this was far from being the case—he had seen
too much of its effects to doubt of its existence, and I
know farther that in some manuscript notes that he
left behind him he had particularly noted the place
which had proved fatal to him as a most unhealthy
one. On enquiring at Boccano early in November, I
found the whole of the people employed about it had
been attacked by the fever this season, several of
them more than once; and it was only within a few
days, I was told, that all the postillions had been at
their post together, since the fever first appeared
among them.

Dr. S. was attacked on his arrival at Florence :—
the debility early in the disease was extreme; no remission occurred, and his stomach was so irritable that

nothing would remain in it—he died on the thirteenth day. Dr. Slaney was a man of the most amiable manners, and much respected by all who knew him. He was a diligent cultivator, too, of that profession of which he formed so worthy a member. Mrs. Slaney was attacked two days after her husband and very narrowly escaped sharing his fate, a slight remission occurred in her case which was taken advantage of, and the bark assiduously administered.

Another English family slept at Baccano on the same night with Dr. Slaney and two of the servants were attacked and one died. Well might the survivors on this melancholy occasion join in the following invective of Domiano in his letter to Pope Nicholas II. (in the eleventh century,)—

Roma vorax hominum domat ardua colla virorum,
Roma ferax febrium necis est uberrima frugum,
Romanæ febres stabili sunt jure fideles—
Quem semel invadunt vix a vivente recedunt.

(No. 11. *Page* 223.*)*

It is not a little gratifying to know that an Englishman by his single exertions was the great mean of bringing about a complete reform in the state of medicine, and of introducing the study of the collateral sciences of Botany and Chemistry in Genoa. The gentleman I allude to was the late Dr. William Batt. Dr. Batt soon after leaving Oxford went to Montpelier, then in high reputation as a medical school, where he obtained his degree. He then visited the different Universities of France, Italy, Germany and Holland. With the advantage of thus examining into the state of medicine at the most celebrated Universities of Europe, and of comparing it with that of his own country, Dr. Batt was well calculated to improve his profession wherever he settled. The state of his health induced him to make choice of Genoa, and the good he did there is justly estimated by the Genoese. He not only reformed the state of medicine, but being appointed professor of chemistry in 1778, he first introduced the study of it at Genoa. He was the first, also, to propose and commence the formation of the Botanic Garden, now containing a fine collection of medicinal plants through the zeal and talents of Professor Viviani. He was also by his writings the great means of overcoming the prejudices against the introduction of the cow pox in Genoa. He was long President of the Medical Society of

Genoa, and enriched its transactions with some excellent papers. He published a pharmacopœia, and
many papers, chiefly in the periodical publications of
the day ; among others, an account of the contagious
fever which raged at Genoa in 1800, during which his
exertions were highly praiseworthy. A list of his
writings is given at the end of a handsome elogium
written by Professor Major. Dr. Batt like every other
man who attempts to improve his profession, and a
stranger too, had doubtless to struggle with many
difficulties. " Les traits de l' envie" says " Professor
Major" (Elogium p. 4.) et de la méchanceté ne l' ont
pas epargné ; mais aussi il a trouvé contre eux un
egide assuré dans l' estime qu' avaient pour lui tous
les justes appreciateurs du vrai merite. Il fut attaqué
par la jalousie ; mais il la désespéra par ses succes :
et sut la mepriser en opposant á ses clameurs la can-
deur de son ame."

Dr. Batt died in February 1812 at the age of 68,
regretted by all ranks of the Genoese : Professor
Major, mentioning his death, concludes with the following high encomium " A peine le bruit de ce mal-
heur se repandit dans le public, que les larmes echap-
paient de tous les yeux, les malades reclamaient leur
Esculape, les pauvres leur appui, leur consolateur;
les hommes de bien l'ont pleuré, et l' envie qui n'avait
point epargné sa renommée est forcée de garder le
silence, et d'honorer meme sa memoire." I make no
apology for the length of this note. Nothing can

surely be more gratifying than to learn and record such traits of conduct of a countryman particularly in a foreign land. To have passed over Genoa without paying my feeble tribute of respect to the memory of so good and meritorious a man, and who was much venerated in the country which he adopted, would have been an injustice.

FINIS.

T. VIGURS, PRINTER, PENZANCE.

Milton Keynes UK
Ingram Content Group UK Ltd.
UKHW032319161024
449665UK00001B/47